Contents

Foreword

There can be no doubt we are in the midst of a revolution in the NHS. The information age is challenging virtually every aspect of what we and it does. In primary care, the last 12 months have seen two significant obstacles overcome – the connecting of GPs to the NHSnet and the legitimisation of electronic records for GPs. We in primary care now have two of the tools we need to begin our path to paperlessness: an infrastructure over which we can begin to communicate electronically, and the freedom to start working with electronic patient records. Such a sea change is not to be underestimated and the many will need to be guided by the few that are there already. Dr Simon Bradley's book recognises that the path to paperlessness is complex and not just confined to computers, e-mail, web browsing or EPRs. The Luddites, obsessives, your staff, your PCG and even the legal eagles need to be brought on board as well. Not intended for the IT-rich, Simon's book is an excellent place for anyone aspiring to the new technologies to start. It is written in a clear non-technical narrative that speaks with the wisdom of an old hand's years of accumulated day-to-day experience. It approaches IT as it should be approached, as a servant for use by the practice. The book covers the full range of issues that any paperless practice will need to consider, in many areas offering sensible practical advice and solutions. For those pondering paperlessness, it is an essential read.

Dr Paul Cundy
General Practitioner
Chairman, IMT Sub-committee of the GPC
Chairman, Joint Computing Group
of the RCGP and the GPC
February 2001

The Paperless Practice

Simon Bradley

General Practitioner, Trainer, IT Beacon Lead
Bristol

Foreword by
Paul Cundy

Chairman
GPC IMT Sub-committee
and Joint Computing Group

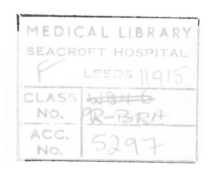
Radcliffe Medical Press

Radcliffe Medical Press Ltd
18 Marcham Road, Abingdon, Oxon OX14 1AA

British Library Cataloguing in Publication Data

A catalogue record for this book is available from the British Library.

ISBN 1 85775 486 7

Typeset by Joshua Associates Ltd, Oxford
Printed and bound by TJ International Ltd, Padstow, Cornwall

Preface

'Dr McCoy to the transporter room' and the subsequent 'beaming up' performed by Scotty are as unreal a choice in today's car-based society as was the Internet and electronic communications at the creation of the NHS a mere 50 years ago. Yet now near instant synchronous visual and auditory communication are possible between a doctor and patient on opposite sides of the world, all for less than the cost of a local-rate phone call. This is a magnitude of change as great as would be the change from the car to the transporter, and primary care is in the front line of that change.

There are more than 175 million people able to go online worldwide. Computers are being given away free with a connection to the Internet. Internet suppliers are providing free telephone calls as well as free access to the Internet. In the USA $48 million dollars was spent in online commerce in 1998–99 and Europe is expected to overtake the USA by 2002. All general practices are to be connected to a computer network for the NHS (NHSnet) by April 2001. We are truly seeing a revolutionary change in the way we live, work and communicate. Changes that are transforming society as would Scotty's transporter, are creating new problems. Just as beaming patients into the consulting room might solve problems, can you imagine what it would mean if patients could bypass your receptionist and materialise in front of you in the surgery every time they sneezed? Unthinkable!

The information revolution threatens many of our traditional ways of working. Whenever there is change, there is opposition to those changes, often reasonably so. It can be very difficult to work out what to keep and what to throw away. The industrial revolution, whilst it brought prosperity, also brought new disease and pollution, so maybe the Luddites were right.

Right or wrong however they could not stand in the path of change and command it to 'stop', and neither can we in general practice resist the inevitability of computerisation and information technology in healthcare. Those who require information from us in electronic form will demand it. The pharmacist will demand electronic prescriptions, the insurance company will demand their electronic PMA reports and our colleagues will demand electronic referrals and summaries that they can integrate with their own records and transmit digitally around their own organisations. Society is changing and we, as part of society, must change too.

This convulsion in the way we work is going to be uncomfortable for most of us. Not only are we going to have to learn new skills, such as how to operate a mouse and type on a keyboard, but we will also have to change our working processes within our practices to get the most out of electronically stored and transmitted information. Whilst on the journey into this new territory we will inevitably, at times, get a bit lost, get things wrong and have to review our position and change direction. What we need to know is how to reduce the risk of things going wrong, learn from the experience of those who have travelled this way before and try to choose the best route first time. This is how this book will seek to help you. By focusing on the clinical and business imperatives within primary care and keeping them squarely in view throughout, the technology becomes seen merely as a tool to improve patient care and the efficient delivery of that care in general practice.

Covering emerging technologies that, at today's oppressive and accelerating rate of change, may soon become tomorrow's standards, it will help to guide you towards the best position to take advantage of new developments. The level of uptake of IT already varies tremendously, so for some the starting point will be not having a computer at all and they may be asking where do we start and how can we catch up? This book will try to show the most effective route. Others in the middle will be making use of computers for prescribing, call and recall and will want to know how to move towards the use of the computer to maintain medical records. This book can help here too. All practices will be looking at how to utilise computers most effectively within primary care groups (PCGs) and with the pressures of clinical governance and cost-effective prescribing. At the same time we all have to cope with the implications of connecting to NHSnet and its associated electronic communications in support of the developing electronic health record. This book can be used as a guide for all of this. It can either be dipped into as the practice extends its computer system and problems arise, or used in a more structured way as a readable handbook to assist the clinician navigating through these interesting times.

Simon Bradley
February 2001

Introduction

First there was funding

The paperless surgery, though currently a relative rarity, is destined to spread and multiply until it effects the whole body of general practice. If we start preparing for it now, treating it as an evolutionary rather than a revolutionary process, then what may seem to many to be a threatening parasite may become a welcome commensal. Apart from the general change of culture, two things in particular are going to accelerate this process. These are the legal legitimisation of the computer record for storing patient medical records in primary care and the connection of all computerised practices to NHSnet, together with the associated, substantial investment in GP computing. It was the presence of financial incentives, direct and indirect, that kicked off the computerisation of primary care in the UK in the late 1980s.

Free computers in return for prescribing data began the widespread computerisation of general practice; enthusiastic practices could start to experiment with computers with little direct cost to themselves. This was accelerated by the 1990 Contract. Its obsession with targets and evidence-less health promotion required morbidity registers and call and recall systems, which could only be managed effectively by computer. Whilst being of questionable benefit to patients, the remuneration of GPs became inextricably linked with these processes.

Finance was once again the prime motivator in the near universal use of computers in general practice with the push for GP/health authority Links for registration and item of service claims. With savings of as much as £150 000 per year possible in a single health authority, reimbursements for GP computer systems rose from the normal 50% to up to 100%. Driven by the benefit for health authorities, the uncomputerised practice has become the exception. This computerisation was, however, limited in its scope of supporting the financial claims processes of GPs and the work could be undertaken in its entirety by non-clinical staff. The GP still did not have to touch the technology.

A horse called EDI

Disguised within the GP/health authority Links business arrangement was the Trojan Horse that would bring the paperless surgery a significant step closer. That horse was called EDI or, to give it its full name, electronic data interchange. This allowed direct communication between disparate computer systems in general practices and health authorities. Health-related information could be incorporated into and used by the receiving computer with minimal human intervention. This put hardware and software into practices to link them to the Racal Health Care network, a communications infrastructure on which future electronic communications within the health service could be based. Within three years 80% of practices were using electronic communications for patient registration, with acceptance of paperless information exchange in the mainstream of general practice. Almost unrecognised, the migration to the paperless practice had commenced.

This first step of communication between different computer systems established UN EDIFACT as the agreed format for healthcare computer communications. This rules-based and rigid standard was between the single Exeter NHS computer system used by all health authorities and a multitude of GP suppliers. It gave a single fixed point at one end of the communications process. The next step was to connect the multitude of GP systems with a further multitude of hospital systems. This was a much more difficult task as it involved dealing with greater variables at both ends, as well as handling clinical information that could impact directly on the care of individual patients – it had to be correct. This process started with the definition of a clinical message standard based again on UN EDIFACT. More important than the standard, however, was the clinical information content definitions and requirements contained within the clinical message. What is a U + E? What are the components of the test? Who defines the normal range? What happens if a flag is attached that says the result is normal? Do we all mean the same thing by 'normal'? Messages for pathology results were successfully piloted in the Avon Trailblazer and became available for national implementation in the autumn of 1998.

Information for Health

Whilst the software and hardware infrastructure of clinical computing was developing, the new Labour Government came into office in May 1997. In its subsequent White Paper, Tony Blair heralded the NHSnet connection project with an undertaking to connect GPs to an NHS information super-highway; Frank Burns was seconded to the Department of Health to produce an information strategy for the NHS, and *Information for Health* was published in September 1998.

> **Box 1** Key objectives of *Information for Health*
>
> - Lifelong electronic health records for every person in the country.
> - Round-the-clock online access to patient records and information about best clinical practice, for all NHS clinicians.
> - Genuinely seamless care for patients through GPs, hospitals and community services sharing information across the NHS superhighway.
> - Fast and convenient access to information and care through online information services and telemedicine.
> - The effective use of NHS resources by providing health planners and managers with the information they need.

It recognised the need for person-based, securely held confidential information, which had to be derived from operational systems. It further recognised that the information so derived would need to support health improvement programmes, primary care groups and clinical governance arrangements, and be available for collaboration and sharing across the NHS and with local authorities; a tall order indeed but one that the Government sees as central to the modernisation of the NHS. It set some specific targets and has now attached dates to some of them which are fleshed out further in *Building the Information Core: implementing the NHS Plan* (http://www.doh.gov.uk/nhsexipu/strategy/update).

Legitimisation of the electronic patient record

Although for years many GPs have maintained an electronic record of patient care they were in fact breaking their terms of service. On 28 September it was announced that from 1 October 2000, GPs could maintain an electronic patient record (EPR) if they so wished. Though this appears to be initial cause for celebration, practices will need to apply and show that they maintain a suitable electronic record system before they can do so legitimately. New practices will need to apply, as will those practices that have been using an EPR system for years. Health authorities will, with help from their LMC, have to decide how to assess whether practices are compliant and will have to appoint an officer in charge of this assessment process. The system must be RFA(99)-compliant to be allowed to use the EPR. It must have audit functions and GPs must sign an agreement that they will not tamper with those security functions and also that they agree to adhere to good practice guidelines in the maintenance of those records. Provided common sense applies in the interpretation of the statutory instrument, this should not stand in many GPs way and, for most practices, will represent a significant milestone on the road to becoming paperless.

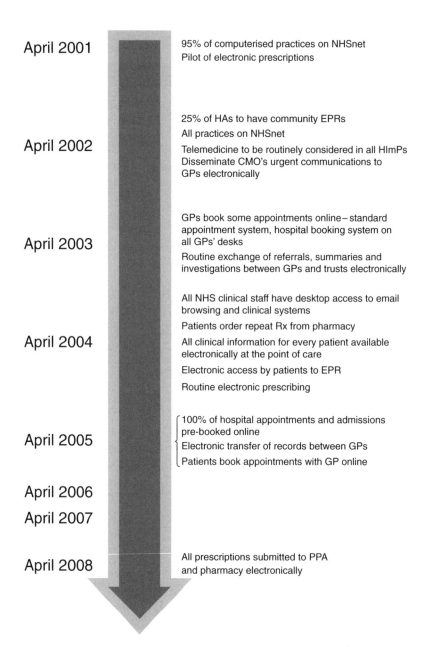

Figure 1 NHS IT timeline.

Figure 1 NHS IT timeline.

1
Lauding the Luddite

Cultural dissonance

Many students entering medicine consider it a vocation where care of the patient is first and foremost. Nowhere is this feeling stronger than for those going into general practice where having an ongoing, face-to-face, personal, medical relationship with patients is of particular importance. It should therefore surprise no one that the cultural dissonance associated with information technology is particularly strong for clinicians in primary care. Boxes that whirr and impersonal screens of text are bad enough without having to learn new skills like typing and how to use a mouse. These interrupt the natural ebb and flow of verbal and non-verbal communication, which is key to the consultation and the doctor–patient relationship. It makes even a battle-hardened technophile like me want to throw the PC out of the window and get on with the real work of caring for patients. Yet the ever-increasing amount of information on patients and their management requires that I am well informed in order to offer a reasonable quality of care. If the information is unavailable, incorrect or inadequate I am at a very real risk of not only getting things wrong but, in these increasingly litigious times, of also being punished for it. Yet I work in a partnership where I rely on my partners and others for many things including the maintenance of patient records, and if we are to move forward we need to be able to share the information we all gather. So we need to move forward together. Can this change be managed and the discomfort of a new way of working minimised? I believe it can, so read on!

In Avon our experience of introducing the electronic transmission of pathology results as part of the national Trailblazer project taught us a great deal about the impact of computerisation on the GP. Many practices were just not ready for it. If the primary function of the computer in your consulting rooms is to support a plant and it is never switched on, having your patients' urea and electrolytes on it 18 hours after their blood is taken is of no value to you. If you do not use the computer then taking on sophisticated clinical messaging is destined to fail. Recovering from failure is far harder than introducing change effectively in the first place. We need to recognise the limits to change imposed by the 'Luddite' streak in our own personalities and those of our partners and colleagues. Recognising the reasons for resisting change, which are often very reasonable, and finding ways for the technology to add value to the consultation as well as introducing change in an incremental, non-threatening way are crucial to implementing change in the practice. This is as true for our partners as it is for the rest of our staff.

Acknowledge anxiety

Take for instance the hypothetical Senior Partner who is five years from retirement and has given 30 years of high-quality personal care to many of your current patients from before they were born. Why should she change? Why should she give up the ability to sketch her findings and read between the ink-scribed lines on a Lloyd George record? Your introduction of change says to her that her care has been inadequate. It is a direct criticism of what she has given her working life to providing. You need to listen to her but not only does she need to be listened to but she must *feel* listened to and must *feel* heard and understood. Use summarisation as you would in a consultation to let her know that her anxieties have been recognised. Agree on the inadequacy of the computer as a medium for the sketch and meet on the common ground of improving medical care of patients. Give her the credit that is due for organising the paper records and systems in the practice and move forward onto how this provides the basis from which records may be more easily put onto the computer. Reinforce the positives. If the practice has seen the value of using the computer as a repeat-prescribing tool, build on that success by starting the computerisation of the consultation with acute prescribing; facilitate your partner's use by setting her default screen to be in the prescribing module. Make it as little effort for her as possible to use the system.

Identify problems and solve them

Consider the layout of the consulting room: how does she consult? How can the computer and printer be organised to disrupt the consultation and desk as little as possible? Does she share the records with the patient or keep them securely clamped to her chest? The former may demand a monitor half turned to the patient and the latter turned firmly away. If the desk is cramped, how about suggesting a wall-mounted sphygmomanometer to gain some space, screwing the printer to the wall or raising both the printer and monitor on an arm so that they can be swung into or out of play. Don't be afraid to use the sexiness of the technology to woo her to its use. A flat (TFT) screen takes up little space, is only slightly more expensive than a traditional monitor and reflects senior partner status. To my knowledge just such a screen was the persuading factor in getting one senior NHS executive to use e-mail!

Does she have a particular clinical interest? Use this interest to show the value of entering coded data in the consultation, even if you have to start with a clerk entering the data for her after the consultation. Things that may at first seem the antithesis of computerisation, such as mental health, can be enhanced by the use of a checklist or template such as the CAGE questionnaire for the individual drinking 24+ units per week, or the use of a depression rating scale in someone who suffers from TATT (Tired All The Time). Mmmm . . . must do one myself when I'm not so tired!

Even if she does not want to enter the data herself, the collection of information by nursing staff can be extracted from the computer and fed back to reward her interest and make her more receptive towards the use of technology to enhance patient care. It is useful to involve the whole team in this thereby strengthening a practice-wide consistent use of information, enhancing the quality of the data and the effectiveness of the use it may be put to, as well as, of course, demonstrating the extra benefit of the computer as a clinical tool to those most resistant to it.

Money is a powerful motivator and, for instance, an onscreen reminder to do a new registration medical can net thousands of pounds when there has been a change of list in the practice, as well as enabling the associated routine screening. The recording of such health promotion advice is going to become increasingly important in ensuring quality practice payments are accrued. For many practices this opportunistic intervention is the most effective way of ensuring health promotion activities are carried out. The common sense in using the computer as a tool to collect information that supports our pay, no matter how clinically relevant or otherwise, will strike a chord with all but the most hardened technophobe and can be used to justify and pay for that sexy new monitor. If that is not enough, the looming national service framework (NSF) for ischaemic heart disease, to name the first of many, is a stick to drive us on.

Other interests, such as research, may be enhanced by access to tools such as Medline, which hugely simplify access to journals and clinical articles. Links can be set up on the partner's desktop so that the single click of a button can take her to the BMJ or RCGP website for latest medical news, or to the *Financial Times* site, so she can check on her share portfolio between patients. If the partner is a trainer, links to other training practices can be a great help. Many publish their registrar tutorials on the web and these can be a relevant and helpful tool for the trainer, e.g. making the individual partner's need, supported by the technology, a single unit: to improve job satisfaction and the extent of use of the computer in the consulting room.

E-mail in the consulting room is a great timesaver for the political partner who is a member of the LMC or PCG, or both, and who is deluged with documents that otherwise would arrive by post on the day of the meeting without time for serious review. Sharing documents with automated revision notes is a boon for the clinical governance GP in the PCG for instance; different colours highlight the new comments on a document and display those comments clearly. You can know who altered what and when and share the benefits of multiple authorship of a single document without the delays of circulating and collating paper. If you or your practice manager knows how to use e-mail, why don't you chase the LMC and PCG to get them on-line? What about the health authority? They must be able to use e-mail. Make sure they have your address, NHSnet and the Internet and tell them to use it. Just as being the only person with a telephone is useless, being the only person on e-mail is too. The more people who use the technology the more useful it becomes and nowhere is this more true than with e-mail. Make the technology work for all partners in the

Table 1.1 Sample form identifying individual interests

Name	Role	Interest	Problem	Solution
Dr Jane Lud	Senior Partner	Finance	Achieving quality practice targets	Design templates that prompt for QP data and a regular audit that feeds back progress to achieving payments
		Maternity care	Women not on folic acid	Add entry to family planning and antenatal template to prompt the user to give folate advice and print off a folate advice leaflet to hand to the patient in the consultation
		Son and daughter (away at university)	They never ring	Get the kids' e-mail addresses and show Jane how to e-mail them. When they reply to say they will be home for her birthday at the weekend, you've won!!
James Dul	CPN	Psychiatry	Part time – does not get to see all GPs every week	In-house e-mail ensures messages are not lost. Turning on a status flag shows when they have been read so he knows the message has been received and noted

Dr Del Udit	Concealed depression	Identifying those presenting for TATT bloods who are depressed	Computerised Hamilton Rating Scale performed by phlebotomist. Score greater than 12 generates referral to James
	Trainer	Training	Impending re-approval	Computerise training log Secretary to construct training library database Get approval pro-forma on disk from Regional Post Graduate Dean
	PCG lead GP	Everything!	Everything!!!	Set up computerised diary shared over the Internet and available to PCG CEO, practice manager and Del Show document electronically, sharing revision and amendment tracking

practice. Use a simple form to identify individual interests and problems they may be having and then use the technology to solve those problems.

Make IT work for everyone

Don't stop with just partners though. The needs of nurses, receptionists and attached staff should all be analysed to see how the technology can be used to improve both the quality of patient care they offer and their job satisfaction. Why don't you get your practice manager to show the health visitor for the elderly how to access Medline and pull down a few articles on falls prevention in the older person, for instance, or your receptionist how to e-mail the health authority for more domiciliary chiropody forms, rather than spending ages waiting on the phone. General, positive feelings towards IT in the practice spread by osmosis through even the hardest meniscus. Soon even the most resistant individual will be benefiting from the technology and asking how to get more from it. Not because they suddenly like IT but because it solves problems that sometimes they did not realise were there in the first place.

Remember your models for helping patients change their behaviour: the ambivalent smoker faced with an overtly persuasive effort to stop who, almost as a reflex, adopts the opposing line? The same goes for your partners and colleagues and computerisation. Faced with 'we should go to paperless consultations' the likely response will be 'No' or 'No because . . .'. Negotiation is the preferred tactic.

We need to move our colleagues through the cycle of change, preparing the ground so that change can be considered. Making the benefits of the technology clear in the contemplation phase, identifying and addressing the risks and establishing how costs will be met are necessary steps in preparing the ground for change. Monetary costs

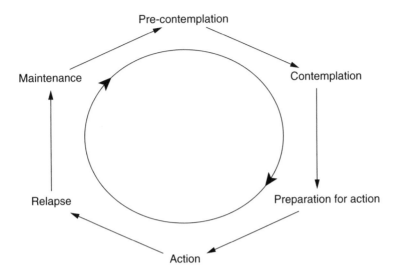

Figure 1.1 The cycle of change.

Source: Prochaska JO and DiClemente CC (1986) Towards a comprehensive model of change. In *Treating Addictive Behaviors* (eds R Miller and N Heather). Plenum Press, New York.

and the time required for training need to be identified, as does how they will be resourced. If expending the resource is inevitable and forces outside of our control are placing the change on us, then this too should be recognised. If the reality that we are all going to be connected to NHSnet and have a computer in the consulting room is recognised, then the reluctant partner will start with this as a fact of life and will be much more prepared to talk about how it can be made to help, not hinder, the work.

As with smoking cessation where getting rid of the ashtrays around the house may be a change in lifestyle that helps the smoker to give up his old ways, the paper-loving partner, having reached the action stage, may need to change other things around them. For instance, on starting to use clinical links, paper and electronic results need to come in parallel for a while; the paperphile will usually need to have her paper blood test results taken from her intray and hidden from view before she will start to use those that come electronically.

A clear goal is needed at this stage, together with an appropriate plan and appropriate rewards. So where the early receipt of results has improved patient care, advertise it. Where values for rubella status and haemoglobin can now be integrated and displayed within the maternity template, demonstrate it. Avoid the risk of relapse by having clear contingency plans in place for when something goes wrong with the electronic system, as it surely will, so that exposure to the old habit is minimised.

The message is clear to the Luddite in us and our practices: concentrate on the clinical and practical benefits of the technology and present the evidence to support the individual interests and working needs of all practice members, and a natural momentum for adopting the new technology will gather so that change management will only need a gentle touch on the tiller.

2
The electronic health record: achieving paperlessness

Information is central to patient care and the better the information we have on our patients' conditions the better our decisions are likely to be, and the better the outcome for the individual patient. There are problems though, even if we collect the correct information. Will it be available to us when we need it and will it be presented in a way that we can quickly make sense of? An envelope stuffed full of pink INR results for the anticoagulated patient can make it impossible to see the full blood count we were really after. It is just this sort of problem that the electronic health record (EHR) seeks to avoid and it is for this reason that the UK Government has set tough targets in its strategy, *Information for Health*, for achieving a lifelong EHR for every person in the country. It also identifies primary care as the key place for the EHR to be held so what we do will have prime influence on the management of all health information.

Our clinical, hospital-based colleagues will input information necessary to their care of the patient but their systems will be required to output it in a format our systems can understand and that we can use. Report requests from solicitors, insurance company risk assessments, faxes from casualty, handwritten notes from patients, discharge letters in, it seems, as many different formats as there are consultant firms, results from X-rays, pathology reports,

ECGs and peak flow forms – over the years a blizzard of paper has become an avalanche that almost threatens to blank out the light. How can we see even the possibility of achieving paperlessness? If we are to get there each of these paper flows will need to be converted to electronic forms. Then, of course, there is verbal communication that must be recorded, and in the consultation, our interpretation of non-verbal cues and the documentation of the results of our physical examination. In reception, information likewise comes by phone, fax, scribbled on the back of envelopes and in person. Our receptionists and administrative staff too must collect, collate, record and share this information with the rest of the team. Where do we start? It seems almost overwhelming.

The beginning

A good place to start: a new patient presents and completes a registration questionnaire and registration form. How does this get onto the clinical system? There is the demographic information – name, address, NHS number and the like as well as the clinical information. Although it would seem sensible for our systems to be able to input just the new ten-digit NHS number, at present the National Strategic Tracing Service does not support online automated query and lookup by GPs. This is still a long way off. So our receptionists will have to do it. Our paper forms completed by the patient should resemble the electronic format entered by our receptionists. If the layout, down to the level of the typeface (font), are the same it helps overcome some cultural disincentives to using the electronic format. If they are in the same sequence on the screen as on the forms as the receptionist's eyes move naturally from field to field, data entry becomes faster and is likely to be more accurate. Simple things make it simple.

The clinical information on the self-completed new patient forms should also follow a logical sequence. Which of the questions we include here should also be checked by the practice nurse or doctor at the new patient medical? Can we capture the information that is relevant to the NSF or HImP or additional information that is required for local research or audit? Use of on-screen form templates facilitate the entry of coded information and speed data entry. Use them whenever a lot of information is to be gathered and it is important not to miss things out. Break information into logical sets and create sub-templates to avoid making the information requirement seem excessive or the screen cluttered.

Information to be added to the EPR has to be made at an access point and does not at this time have the portability of the paper record, though wireless access may give mobile data entry points in the future. So we have to think about the physical points of data entry. In reception this means that we need an access point at the place that information is captured or viewed. This may be a dumb terminal or PC (I will call them terminals from now on) – dumb or intelligent as you see is appropriate to your needs. One is needed at the front desk at least, as appointments are viewed, prescription queries checked and minor address changes made at the point that the patient is greeted in the surgery. The other place that a terminal is needed is where the practice phone is answered, as the same issues arise here as when the patient is physically present and so the same facility for information access is needed.

Variety may be the spice of life but in practice presenting information in a predictable way decreases the requirement for training, as less additional knowledge is required to enter or access information. Dumb terminals restrict use but, as there is less to go wrong, require less maintenance and support. Why choose a PC where there is no requirement to use the additional functions it can offer? If you do use a PC, think about offering a restricted set of applications presented as a standard set-up for that location. This often increases confidence in users as they become familiar with the restricted function set that meets their requirements. At reception this may well just mean access to the clinical system and internal e-mail.

In the office the need to access additional information increases and a PC will almost certainly be needed. Just what do you require your secretary to be able to do? This information will govern the feature set she will need. She will need to type letters, take dictation or transcribe from tape, answer queries from patients and from clinicians inside and outside the practice, enter coded data into the clinical system, perhaps from incoming letters, and track non-NHS letters, forms and reports. Will she need to enter scanned data? The list goes on and requires an increasing and high degree of training.

A checklist of who uses particular software and for what purpose helps to identify where issues and training needs arise (*see* Table 2.1).

It is therefore vital to commence with key areas, train and then add to them to build on knowledge and not overwhelm everyone with too many choices. Go for low-hanging fruit and enable as many people as possible to pick them. Things as relatively simple as pop-up messaging or internal e-mail can have tremendous benefits to the working lives of administrative staff in the practice. It is as immensely frustrating for the receptionist to wait outside the surgery door as it is for the GP to be interrupted when he has a patient with him. A pop-up message that appears in real time (or as it is sent) saying that there is an important call or that a patient has arrived late and is demanding to be seen NOW!, can save the receptionist time and allow you to decide whether the urgency is one that warrants interruption of your current consultation. It is simple technology but it works.

Table 2.1 Software checklist

Type	Wordprocessor
Transcribe	Voice management software
Fax	Computer fax software
Access clinical system	Clinical system familiarity
Enter coded data	Read Code expertise . . . currency and active problem management
Scan data	Scanning and OCR software
Workflow tracking	Spreadsheets
Financial management	Accounts software
Payroll	Payroll software
Appointments	Clinical appointment system
Issue repeat prescriptions	Clinical system prescribing module
Search	Extract data for PCT/health authority
E-mail	E-mail client software
Internet	Rail times/order/purchase
Back-up	Tape software and procedures
EDI	Pathology and radiology results, pathology requesting with discharge and upcoming referrals
Rostering	On-call/rooms/holidays
Web-site management	HTML software
Newsletter production	DTP software
Research	Database software
Pop-up messaging	Clinical system or add on

3
E-mail

Everyone has become familiar with e-mail over the last few years, even if it is just to recognise the e-mail address quoted at the end of every consumer programme on the television. For most GPs, just how this new form of communication should be used to its greatest effect is often a matter of trial and error. This chapter will give a few ideas on how we can use e-mail to improve communication within and between practices.

The fax allowed us to take a paper document and distribute it to others with the immediacy provided by the phone, but it was not until the widespread presence of fax machines in virtually every practice and hospital department that it gave us real value from the technology. Similarly, e-mail only becomes really useful when a critical mass of those we wish to communicate with are using it. In primary care that critical mass is here now! So start using it and as you do so the benefits will accrue (*see* Box 3.1).

E-mail in-house

Some practice systems have an e-mail facility within the clinical system. The familiarity that use of the practice system brings means that all staff can quickly gain competence with this usually pretty basic e-mail facility. It also means that systems with dumb terminals can support e-mail and you don't have to have PCs on every desk and a

---

Box 3.1 Benefits of e-mail

- Immediate transmission of your message.
- You always keep the original message, you send just a copy.
- Ability to broadcast your message to *all* those to whom you wish to send it.
- Easy forwarding of messages.
- Automatic inclusion of quotes from received e-mail.
- The ability to collect your mail wherever you are.
- The ability to send a message to someone who is not actively logged on to the computer system or the Internet.

---

practice-wide network. Yet even simple e-mail rapidly proves its worth, with staff and partners able to send messages to other members of the team who are not at their desk. This quickly replaces the sticky post-it notes stuck on desks and notes folders, and so another unnecessary piece of paper bites the dust.

Similarly, e-mail can replace the practice's message book. Instead of handwritten messages squeezed together on a page that always seems too small and where it is all too easy for one to be overlooked, the electronic version goes directly to the person to whom it was intended and, what's more, the sender can usually check that it has been read. Automatic time and date stamping and the use of log-on passwords and audit trails improve the security of in-house messaging, and the days of the denial 'I didn't get the message' are numbered. Automatic forwarding of mail can ensure that urgent mail is routed to another doctor when one partner is away, and important documents should no longer be left languishing in the bottom of an intray in a distant office.

E-mail and the world

Electronic mail to outside the practice becomes a bit more complicated and requires a connection between a computer within the practice and an outside network. The provider of this connection, where the e-mail in question is to be sent over the Internet, is known as an Internet service provider (ISP). As well as offering certain ISP functions for the health service, NHSnet is a private network (Intranet) of computers provided for the NHS, which allows access to the wider Internet through secure 'gateways'. This allows the transmission of e-mail to the Internet but restricts prying, electronic eyes from getting sight of the confidential patient-based information we keep on our NHS systems. It must be asked, though, how private is private when this Intranet is for the biggest employer in Europe with hundreds of thousands of access points at tens of thousands of sites? So our software, modems and ISDN routers must have security mechanisms to prevent unauthorised access from both within and without the NHS.

Modems and ISDN routers are the hardware that converts the information we wish to send into a form that can be sent over the telecommunications network, and that can then be converted back into something you and I can understand at the other end. These are the windows we open to look out but which can allow others to look in if we are not constantly vigilant. In Chapter 13, confidentiality, security and stopping unwelcome intrusion will be explored in more depth.

Addressing too becomes more complicated when we open ourselves to the Internet and therefore the world. We want to be sure that we get the mail intended for us and therefore there needs to be a unique address for every person using e-mail on the Internet. Sorting out the processes that manage Internet addressing is a massive task but one that need not concern us, the humble user. All that we should need is an ISP such as Demon, BT or even NHSnet for that matter, who will allocate us an address such as nargual.paul@btinternet.com. This is a text address that makes sense to us but really represents a unique number that identifies Dr Paul's mailbox at BT Internet to the world. When Dr Paul dials into his mailbox or you dial into your ISP and you wish to collect your post, a series of passwords log you into your electronic mailbox and downloads any mail in your mailbox into your intray. Your software then sends any mail you have put in your out-tray to your ISP and thence to the intended recipient's mailbox at their ISP. The software to do this usually comes free with the software supplied by your ISP. Internet Explorer, for instance, contains a competent e-mail management software package called Outlook Express. This sort of software is known as an e-mail client and most of these free e-mail clients have bigger siblings with more sophisticated functions for which you have to pay.

The really useful addressing that we are familiar with in terms of telephone directories does not exist for the Internet. There is no central list of e-mail addresses on the net and no system for tracking when people change their address or ISP. There are e-mail registers which attempt to do this of which the largest is Bigfoot (http://www.bigfoot.com) but you have actively to seek them out to join and use them. The big search engines like Yahoo (http://www.yahoo.co.uk) and Excite (http://www.excite.com) are more like Thompson's and Yellow Pages, and locate websites on the Internet by subject rather than name, although they do have quite reasonable e-mail location facilities. The development of a directory for NHSnet is one of its biggest potential advantages over the Internet but its effective development is also one of its biggest challenges. Until there is a comprehensive register, one of the easiest ways to find someone's e-mail address is to give them a call and ask! If you are sent an e-mail, just clicking the 'Reply to' function usually gives you the option of adding that new address to your personal address book, as well as making it easy for you to respond.

E-mail management software not only does the bread and butter of logging us into our mailbox and picking up and sending our post but it also does smart things like flagging mail for degrees of urgency and importance, offering opportunities to remind us to reply. By displaying e-mail by, for instance, date, sender or topic, we can organise this electronic post as we would prefer, in a way that is difficult if not impossible with its paper predecessor. Many programmes allow messages to be colour-coded by sender, so those from the PCG could be in red and those from the health authority in yellow, allowing you at a glance to see which you might consign to the rubbish bin (only joking health authority!).

Advanced e-mail

Increasing sophistication in e-mail programs allows a lot of add-on features to facilitate electronic communication, make them more secure and integrate them with other programs.

E-forms

These are methods of sending structured information. Within Microsoft Outlook, for instance, a task request e-form can be used to assign a task to someone else. This leaves a copy of the request on your 'to do' list and makes a similar entry on the 'to do' list of the person who accepts it. For instance, at a practice meeting the Practice Manager is charged with ensuring that the new hypertension protocol is completed before the next meeting with the senior treatment room Sister responsible for it. The Practice Manager creates

Box 3.2 Do's and don'ts of e-mail

Do:

- consider e-mail overload and only send what is necessary to whom it is necessary
- check your e-mail regularly. There is no point in speeding the process if you only check your mail once a week
- answer immediately if an answer is necessary and you can make a sensible response
- keep it simple:
  - short sentences and paragraphs make quoting in replies easier
  - use plain text (ASCII format)
  - wrap lines after 72 characters
- use the * symbol to emphasise words and text *
- put the subject matter in the header. This is often a matter of just pressing the 'Reply to' button in your e-mail client (e.g. Microsoft Outlook Express)
- be consistent
- delete the original e-mail when replying unless it clarifies your reply
- sign your e-mail
- pause and read all e-mail before sending it.

Remember:

- you can slander and defame as easily electronically as on paper
- out of practice e-mail should not contain patient-identifiable information
- it is easy to seem rude on e-mail so observe normal social conventions unless you actually want to be rude!
- establish rude intent before sending a vitriolic reply
- send text as Rich Text Format with file extension .rtf
- agree a common format for attachments within your PCG
- keep it simple.

Don't:

- use techno babble and abbreviations. These can, IMHO (In My Humble Opinion), irritate and impede communications, although a smiley ☺ or ;-) can make humour obvious and reduce the risk of causing offence
- overdo quotes from the original e-mails
- send uncompressed graphics and images. ISPs may block files over a certain size; they can take forever to download and make you unpopular
- use an automatic signature that gives information that you do not wish to be in the public domain e.g. your home address
- DON'T SHOUT . . . convention has it that capitalised words are the electronic equivalent of shouting.

the e-form entering a date for completion and the degree of urgency associated with it and sends it over the practice network to Sister. Sister receives it and accepts the task. This acceptance is automatically notified to the Practice Manager and recorded on her task list. As Sister gets stuck into diagnosis and investigation she records the work as being 50% complete. Automatically, the Practice Manager is notified of this progress and can inform the impatient clinical governance partner that work is well under way. These forms can be used across the Internet as well as in-house and should prove a boon to the hard pressed PCG lead GP who is juggling more tasks than The Great Alzoomah!

Mailing lists

Software allows potential recipients to be grouped together so that mail can be sent to multiple individuals at the press of a button. When most of our patients are on the web in a year or two the practice e-zine, an electronic practice newsletter, will become a real possibility. It offers more possibilities than a paper magazine, as by tailoring the content to the needs of particular groups we can, for example, send information on sexual health to young people and the new elderly person's fall prevention clinic can be sent to our patients who are over 65 – we can even accompany it with a personal reminder to get a flu jab. When every television is a window on the Internet this will become the norm for our communication with patients. It is coming and you read it here first!! Your PCG should already be sending minutes for board meetings in this way, as well as its quarterly newsletter. Your PCG isn't, I hear you say? Well, give them a kick because it's easily done.

Security and confidentiality

The Internet both opens up a new world of communication and exposes us to a new world of dangers. When we receive e-mail we want to be confident it has not been tampered with en-route, and that it comes from whom it purports to have been sent. When we send e-mail we want to be confident it has been received. This concept is ages old, going back to seals and sealing wax but that's how we want our electronic mail now, signed, sealed and delivered. Software can add digital signatures so you know that it was me who sent you your post. Encryption can keep it for your eyes only. Receipt reports can almost invisibly notify you when the mail is delivered and can even tell you when it has been read.

Box 3.3 Signed, sealed and delivered

If patient-identifiable information is sent anywhere outside of the practice then all three strictures should apply. Sign it (digitally), seal it (encrypt) and make sure it has been delivered by attaching a requirement for a receipt report.

Attachments

No that's not how you feel about your old roll top desk, which hasn't room for a printer. An attachment is a digital object that can be stuck on to your e-mail which, when clicked on with the mouse, can open up to reveal a spreadsheet of your increased list size and decreased visits! Well, we all live in hope. Attachments are anything that can be stored in electronic format; programs, photos, spreadsheets, calendars, webpages, documents in all their many styles, forms, in fact just about anything we currently see on paper and more besides. Sounds and even video can be transmitted as attachments.

It's easy to add an attachment too. You simply click on the paper clip icon on your e-mail program, or click 'Attach' in the appropriate menu, browse to find the relevant file and click on 'OK'. In the Microsoft Office family of products, if you are working on the file you wish to send, you can click on 'Send to' in the 'File' menu and it automatically brings up the choice of sending it by e-mail and boots the appropriate software. Just as with e-mail, when you send an attachment you do not physically lose what you send. Only a copy is sent and the original remains secure for future use on your hard drive. Here are some hints about attachments:

- do compress large attachments – watch out for images, which can be huge

- do not open attachments from anyone you don't know

- do identify the attachment file type and content in your covering e-mail.

Box 3.4 Dangerous attachments

Attachments may be virus carriers. These do no harm if they are just downloaded but if they are opened or executed they can replicate and damage your computer. Even some documents can carry viruses; for instance, Microsoft Word documents can have macro viruses. Melissa, one of the first of these, was little more than a nasty dose of flu that you gave to all your friends. Unfortunately, macro viruses have undergone something akin to antigenic shift and are much more virulent. They can do serious harm and mail themselves with a tantalising message, such as 'I love you', to everyone in your address book.

Always have an up-to-date virus checker on any PC connected to a network or the Internet.

Signatures

It is easy to automatically add detail that is of a repetitive nature, like your signature, phone and fax number and maybe your web address, to the bottom of every e-mail you send. You create a 'signature' in your e-mail program that is stored as a text file. You can set it to be appended to every outgoing piece of mail. It is useful information but if your signature contains your home phone number you might not want it to be appended to e-mails to your patients. Some people add 'amusing' by-lines to their signatures that, in true Victor Meldrew mode, get right up my nose. But more than just irritating, these might be harmful if appended to an e-mail to a patient as they could easily be taken out of context (Figure 3.1).

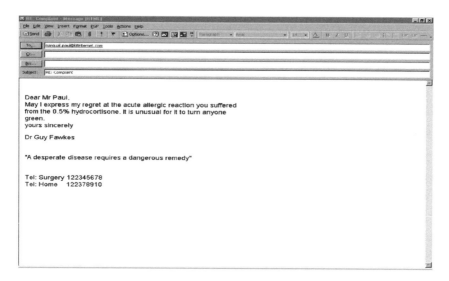

Figure 3.1 A potentially dangerous attachment!

Burnt spam

I'm not talking about tins of the insipid, synthetic, condensed meat so beloved of Monty Python but just as their choice of spam, eggs and spam, spam sausage and spam and even spam, spam and spam, meant that spam came with everything, spam is unavoidable on the Net. Junk e-mail, advertising and get rich quick promotions land on your electronic doormat just like those unwanted flyers do at home. When you get spammed the best approach is to just delete it without reply. If it continues then a request to be taken off the mailing list is the most you should respond. Some e-mail programs have spam filters, which dump the unwanted gloop in a background file for you to peruse briefly before binning. There are some specific anti-spam programs available, which look for spam in your inbox at your ISP and delete it before you download onto your PC. One such program you might like to try is Spam Eater Pro, available on trial at http://www.hms.com. Commercial spam is not allowed on NHSnet but it can still be sent from outside.

Flame mail

Flaming is the vitriol that is poured on you if you upset someone by e-mail and is the unpleasant, offensive content in an e-mail. It is all too easy for the technology to send a stream of such flame mailings that can bring the receiving system to its knees and even, on occasion, stop it functioning altogether. Hopefully, this won't happen in the medical community too often but careful adherence to the e-mail advice given previously can reduce the possibility of being flamed.

There is no doubt that e-mail is one of the most useful

tools of the information revolution. It can enhance the working of all businesses. In the healthcare business this should mean more efficient practices. With up-to-date information that is both more confidential and available than was previously possible with paper, it will mean improved care for patients. It is undoubtedly one of the first places to start the process of building the paperless practice.

4
Primary care groups

OK guys . . . two things. Two things to remember and repeat mantra-like whenever asked for data by the primary care trust (PCT). From *The New NHS*:

The needs of patients **not** institutions will be at the heart of the New NHS.

From *Information for Health*:

Management information will be derived from operational systems (i.e. those systems that directly support patient care).

Why should we need to memorise these extracts from two of the major documents that direct the NHS and its strategy? PCGs are changing, mutating, a process of shift not drift into PCTs and they will demand more. More information, more data, more evidence to judge performance. Driven by clinical governance, terrified of another Shipman they will demand facts that they can use to say that they have 'managed' appropriately and ensured quality . . . so 'It ain't our fault!' when something goes wrong. They know that heads will roll unless they can show evidence of adequate management. So they will want to collect evidence even when they are not entirely sure why it is being collected: more is better. I say this because this is what happens in bureaucracies and the larger the organisation becomes, so the bureaucracy increases. So remember the yardstick against which all request for information must be judged;

it should be derived from operational systems that put the needs of patients before those of institutions.

The first thing in building an effective paperless information system in the practice in this new world where two legs good, four legs better becomes four legs good, two legs better, is to reduce the information collection to that which is genuinely necessary to improve patient care. Do what is evidence based and keep focused.

Supporting clinical care

Now at least we know where to start when faced with HImPs, clinical governance, NSF targets and performance management. Does the information support the care of the individual patient?

We need good quality information to be able to offer the right treatment options and assist the patient in the perplexing environment of personal health risk management. If we do not know the patient's past history, we don't know what has been tried, what worked and what failed. If we don't have access to the patient's allergies, we risk a severe reaction with our prescription. This is true of LGE (Lloyd George Envelope) or XML (extensible mark-up language; I think I will change my name to Simon bRadley!). This sort of information is the rock upon which GP clinical systems are founded and is there in them all. So we don't need flashy new systems to get the basic information for care right, we just need to use them more effectively. (Though flashy new systems may offer richer information, images, sound, even video, as well as tools for more rapid information entry.) PCGs can collate this information from our operational patient centric systems (EMIS, TOREX etc) for service management and clinical governance. What this requires of us is that we enter patient information in a systematic way. Many GPs already do this well but most could do it better and will be required to do it better still to improve patient care.

Here are another two things to remember, as they will have far-reaching importance: consistency and coding. These are crucial for ensuring high-quality information and through that clinical care of the patient. And don't forget the NSF is upon us!

Consistency and coding

Coding

Coding is important because we need to be able to track information over time, and coded information is searchable. Yup, I know that current technology allows for free text searching but then, although we can find the word or phrase, we lose its context and therefore its meaning. Let's take ischaemic heart disease. We want to find all those patients who have ischaemic heart disease so we can check they are on aspirin if appropriate. So using a free text search we check for all those of our patients who have ischaemic heart disease in their record. The search then pulls up every occurrence of the words and makes no allowances for the fact that the entry is actually 'no history of ischaemic heart disease' or 'family history of ischaemic heart disease' or even 'coronary angiography: ischaemic heart disease not present'. So coding information helps preserve context and therefore meaning.

Consistency

Increasingly, we now share care both within our practices and with outside organisations such as hospital and community trusts. We therefore need to use at least some of our terminology in the same way. We ourselves may use the same term in different ways even when talking about the same patient. So there needs to be some consistent use of the language of patient care within the practice. For example, in the care of the diabetic patient that involves the nurse and GP in the surgery, the district nurses who also may share care and the ophthalmologist, nephrologist and diabetologist. (So we should be generologists!)

In practices we should be striving for two levels of consistency. One I call vertical consistency, that is to use the same term in the same way in the individual patient's record so at least we can keep track of the care of the individual's illness accurately. We need to be aware of the terms used in a patient's record and if a diagnosis and therefore disease description changes, record it as a changed diagnosis. The other is horizontal consistency, which is harder still to achieve; to use language consistently between different patients and different clinicians, so when I use the term 'depression' you understand what I mean. This common understanding helps improve vertical consistency, as we are less likely to choose differing terms when we mean the same thing. This is difficult because it requires communication, debate, compromise and agreement. These all take time and getting agreement out of a group of GPs is always going to be difficult. We have already self-selected our specialty where independent, individual decision making is a core feature. There is no time to lose; we need to start the discussions right now over the clinical terms we intend to use for the common major medical conditions, if we are to agree within the timescales imposed on us.

Right then, back to PCGs and the paperless practice. To improve patient care we need to record information accurately which will ensure good care for our patients where different clinicians deliver that care. Agreed? If PCGs want to aggregate that information it's up to them to extract it from (remember?) our operational systems. So, it's their job. We facilitate it by providing coded consistent information, which benefits our patients. We can also extract information better because of this and as most of us entered practice not just because we are ornery but also because we want to care for our patients to the best of our ability, this is something that will add value to our practice. We should use PCG administrative and technical staff to get information we can use from our systems, package it and present it in the way we want to enhance care in our own practices. I mean who wants to know about MIQUEST and run a query . . . you would have to be a geek!

MIQUEST

OK, so you want to know about MIQUEST? Well, this is going to be high level, as I wouldn't want you thinking I'm a geek. MIQUEST is a medical structured query language that works on different systems to extract and collate information. It is the national chosen solution for getting information out of the major GP systems. For most audits and queries of GP systems the integral search facility present within most clinical systems is fine. It can give us the information we need quickly and uses a familiar interface. The information can then usually be uploaded into a commercial spreadsheet program such as Excel to produce clear tables and pretty graphs that communicate complex information almost at a glance. MIQUEST is a different beast; you have to design the query, create the necessary permission on the GP system and then run the query. It then outputs the query result to a floppy disk, anonymised if you want, which can then be uploaded again into MIQUEST and compared with output to similar queries conducted on other GP systems. Crucial to its effective use is the design of the query but more crucial still for getting something worth having is asking the right question of people who have considered that they might be asked the question in the first place. If the data is not coded in the system, information is not consistently entered, and the same condition is not described in the same way, interpretation is pretty nigh impossible.

This is far from saying what MIQUEST does is not useful, but there is no doubt that competitiveness within and between practices drives us to improve performance. And MIQUEST can enable us to do this across different clinical computer systems. Comparative data is not only interesting, it is vital for getting some idea about how we are doing compared with others and if we are way out of line, why. Is it us, a bug in our patients or a bug in our systems? All of this is important to know. We just need to know why the question is being asked before it is asked and have some idea, even if that idea is wrong, about the likely outcome of the query and what possible actions we might take with it.

MIQUEST can also extract information in much more sophisticated ways than standard GP system searches. For instance, it can pull out all consultations with a particular diagnosis that have produced a particular prescription. Useful information occasionally, but very useful, very occasionally.

MIQUEST as 'The National Solution' also offers the benefit of having someone local with specialist knowledge on how to get good quality information out of our systems. We do not have to know how to do it, just what questions we would like answered and a decision within our practices to enter accurate, consistent, patient information. I would advise the practice to find out who your local MIQUEST geek is and ask them a few questions you think you might like the answers to. Let them run the query, then look at the outcome and think about the serious questions you might like answered in the future. Start agreeing within and without the practice how you intend to use our colourful and varied medical terminology. A great place to start if you're thinking about this is with PRIMIS. Oh no, another bloody acronym? Does the 21st century practice need another acronym? No of course not but you do need PRIMIS.

PRIMIS

PRIMIS has done some of the work for you. Too good to be true? A MIQUEST geek who can get more clinical information from your computer than you ever wanted to know and now PRIMIS has done some of the work for you. PCTs, PCGs, they're brilliant. Now, now don't go over the top. PRIMIS has done some of the additional work you are being asked or going to be asked to do. Giving with one hand, taking some of it back with the other!

PRIMIS, whatever it means, has its roots in CHDGP (Collecting Health Data for General Practice). Aah, those two magic letters 'GP'. This is and was a GP-led project to improve the way data was entered (collected) in, you've guessed it, general practice and as such is inevitably rooted in common sense and pragmatism. A number of general practices under the auspices of Nottingham University, and fertilised with NHS Executive funding, looked at how GPs use data and how this could be improved. It talked about consistency and Read Codes and GP systems and patient management and was then left until it almost died a death. However, after a trailer load of fertiliser it has sprouted as PRIMIS (it's another of those . . . don't you know? PRIMary care Information Services). Its function is as 'a training and support system to make best use of [GP] clinical computer systems'. That is the large print but the slightly smaller print says that it is necessary for the Government's modernisation programmes in clinical governance, performance and NSFs. So it's a melding of external performance management tools with enhancement of practice-based information use through support and training that will enable improved care and produce the evidence to prove it has taken place. No bad thing in my book IF it's done right (note the big if).

PRIMIS will train our PCG/PCT facilitators with a focus on:

- information management skills for primary healthcare teams, so more than just GPs. Hooray!!
- clinical data recording methods
- assessing and improving data quality
- use of MIQUEST
- analysis and interpretation of primary care data
- facilitation and change management.

It's our job as GPs to subvert MIQUEST as a performance management tool and use it within our practices for what it was designed, to improve patient care by identifying what is done well and what could be done better. Grab the people from PRIMIS and use them to train all our staff on how to improve our use of information. The Nottingham experience of the tender shoot of CHDGP was extremely positive; an invigorating experience to be propagated – so we must make sure that the new fertiliser does not turn a potential fruiting vine into a triffid. Let the PRIMISians come with armfuls of suggested clinical terms for use in the NSFs and we can choose the ones that meet the needs of our patients in our operational systems. We must use it to improve the content of our medical records and through that the care of the patient – therein lies an ample harvest.

Read on about . . .

Read Codes, how could I leave these out? I couldn't and believe me I tried. The first thing to know is what Read Codes aren't. They are not codes, not in the true sense. They are in fact a thesaurus of clinical terms. This gives them body and bouquet but like a fine wine they would probably be described entirely differently by two equally expert sommeliers. That's the problem, their very flexibility blurs the precision of use by the average GP (which, most certainly, includes me). They are merging with the American SNOMED classification, so hopefully this hybridisation will make the Codes more vigorous. What follows is a very brief canter through Read Codes.

Read Codes are, as I have said, an extensive list of clinical terms, so much so that they could be used to produce a fully coded electronic medical record with coding for occupation, social information and medication as well as signs, symptoms and diagnosis. They are mapped to other major coding systems such as ICD10 so can be used in secondary as well as primary care. As they have evolved from the original system derived by ex-GP James Read and have been purchased by Her Majesty's Government as the coding system for the NHS, they have several different incantations. Read 4 byte, i.e. comprised of four digits, Read 5 byte comprised of five digits and the latest and greatest, even if least used, Read 3. The bite here is that Read 3 is the latest but has been called 3 and has five digits!! Confused? Well don't be because all you really need to know is the expansion of the code or, in normal speak, the clinical term. So select tinnitus (clinical term) and the system records F583 (code) but you see tinnitus. Clever, eh? This information is then searchable and allows for improved storage, retrieval and analysis of data. The different Read Codes now match pretty accurately to one another too so the version you have is decreasingly important – but of course intercourse with SNOMED may change all this.

Box 4.1 Some hints on Read Codes

- NOS means 'not otherwise specified' . . . err . . . try not to use it, there should be a better alternative.
- Use a code that starts with a letter (A–S are best) for problem titles . . . they represent diagnoses (some GP systems enforce the use of codes starting with letters as problem titles. Select this if you can).
- Codes that begin with R are uncertain or working diagnoses to be used where a definitive diagnosis has yet to be made.
- Try to associate a diagnostic code with its respective investigations, prescription etc, especially where multiple problems are entered. It is confusing to have a problem heading of Genital Herpes with a prescription for amoxycillin and an ear swab!
- *History of* codes are found within Read but confuse the hell out of me. Pneumonia 1993 seems a far more appropriate way of recording information than *history of pneumonia*, so I would say avoid these too.
- Agree the root code you will use and then be as specific as possible when you make a new coded entry, e.g. the practice agrees to use code C10 for diabetes mellitus but when you see a patient with diabetic neuropathy you use the code C106 which is diabetes mellitus plus neuropathy. All searches for the former will include the latter and you never know when you will need the finer level of granularity.

Local implementation strategies

Information for Health was set out to be a national policy for local implementation; to ensure that the Government's will contained in the White Paper was effectively enacted, health authorities had to have local implementation strategies (LIS) in place by March 2000. These local plans detail how resources are to be spent on the delivery of health information systems in the context of other issues such as HImPs and clinical governance. Management boards with stakeholder representatives are required to use the plans to ensure that spending from the health informatics stream of the Modernisation Fund is effective and appropriate, and that the objectives of *Information for Health* are met. This means that any projects that are implemented locally should be consistent with the local strategy. It is therefore very important that the GP stakeholder either directly or through the LMC and PCG provides a consistent articulate counter to the demands of the secondary care services, who are often better able to put together neatly packaged and higher profile informatics projects for consideration by the LIS management board. If you have not been sent a copy of your own, LIS is available at http://www.doh.gov.uk/nhsexipu/ implemen/flis/libindex.htm. This is where the budget is held, so we all need to have a look and then have a say!

Sequestered within the body of the LIS is another organisation that has considerable potential to affect the way we manage our practice information systems. That is the requirement to form local health informatics services (HIS would you believe!). These are real or virtual organisations formed to maximise the local health informatics skills. It is a requirement of *Information for Health* that there is skill sharing across organisational boundaries within the NHS. These have the potential to become bodies that centralise support for our IT infrastructures such as our networks and provide education and training to all those organisations under its umbrella. Few could argue with the logic of such skill sharing. However, we need to be wary of centralisation forming a discrete bundle of HIS, which could result in a remote and unresponsive service working at the speed of the slowest and to the needs of the most powerful stakeholder. Virtual organisations where there is a central point for skill sharing and co-ordination of service provision carry most of the benefits without the potential risk of GPs being the Cinderella who does not get to go to the ball.

5
Clinical messaging: EDI rides again

The nice thing about standards is, there are so many to choose from.
(Ken Olsen)

In many ways Ken defined the problem. There are just too many standards, leaving us not knowing which one to choose. The NHS chose for us and they chose EDIFACT. Now most people know Eddie as the rather slow, difficult chap, who does not work, from the Archers. There are those who say that this is not far wrong when describing the EDI from EDIFACT. E stands for Electronic, D for Data and I for Interchange and the rest is 'For Agriculture Commerce and Trade' and that's FACT! EDI is the transfer of computer readable information in a way that preserves meaning between different computer systems, a sort of Esperanto for, in this case, NHS computer communications. The problem is that the rest of EDIFACT's title is 1988, so although EDIFACT may have been the right horse for 1988, the question arises, is it still the right horse to back 12 years later? The answer would probably be no but as you are the jockey and the race has started, the question becomes how can I make the best of where I am and are there advantages to be gained from being on this horse? Well, a one-word answer to the latter question is 'yes'. I will try to explain why and help you with the former in the following paragraphs.

The first question that arises is why do we need standards. Well, the answer to that is because there are many different GP computer systems and many different systems within many different hospitals. They are used in many different ways for many different things but all relate to one another in some way. OK, so throw them all away and replace them with a single system. That requires a system to look after more than 55 million people who access the NHS in excess of four times each a year, operated by potentially a million different people. That's a heck of a lot of communication. A single central system to cope with this would be massive (and expensive) and any problem would bring the NHS to a halt. And which government worth its electorate would put all its eggs in such a cavernous single basket? So, you have distributed systems with common communication and so as not to incur risk you choose a proven (out of date) system, EDIFACT. It does, however, work.

Your local laboratory puts a creatinine and electrolyte result for Clarrie Grundy into the EDIFACT message and squirts it down Racal or NHSnet. It is picked up by the GP system, which recognises it as Clarrie Grundy's result, recognises it's a C + E, recognises the normal range and the attached text message from the biochemist and places it in your intray to read when you come in in the morning. At the click of a button you can see the results, at another bring up the full clinical record or add a note for action, or file the result in the EPR. It's quick, easy, efficient and here today brought to you reliably by that old horse, EDIFACT. So that's the advantage – we have a tool *today* that improves the way we can look after our patients and run our practices.

Making the best of EDIFACT is not nearly as stupid as it sounds because choosing the message standard to back is the easy bit. Whichever is chosen now, it will develop, change and be replaced by something else. Expect it. The difficult bit is agreeing what goes in the message and what we mean by it and how we can use it when we get it. So it's more about the structure of the message and the content than the message standard and how we use information when we receive it. The beauty of standard messaging is its structure. We can use it to change the way we manage our patients. If every cholesterol we take is automatically entered into our EPR we enter every BP we can. Then at the click of a button we identify those at a high risk of death from occlusive arterio-vascular disease. We can concentrate our efforts on them, rather than flailing around chucking health promotion at all those people who don't need it.

Enough of that, here is how it can be done. Let us assume that our laboratory can send the messages, that we are using NHSnet to receive them, that it works reliably and that we have a system that is capable of receiving those results and processing them in a sensible way. No I'm not dreaming – there are many practices in several different areas of the country that are doing just this, mine included. How do we manage information delivered in this way and what are the benefits, both immediate and potential, that messaging can bring us? With paper we have some sort of intray where we look at our post usually on a daily basis. By the time it arrives with us it has been stamped with a date and a check box of potential tasks to be performed with that piece of paper. Before that, the envelopes containing these messages were opened and sorted into piles for the respective GP or nurse intray. With electronic messages the patient identifiers and the recipient address details are structured so we no longer need a receptionist to sort the messages. The system identifies them and puts them in the electronic equivalent of your intray; not only that, it sorts the results by patient. You have all the incoming results for that individual patient in a bunch. So, no longer do you see a U + E and add an action note and then 20 minutes later discover a liver function test for that patient that changes your earlier action. You can flick through all the results and base the appropriate decision on fuller information. OK, sometimes results come in at different times because of batch processing of the more unusual investigations by the laboratory, but this is much less common. Not only have you saved considerable clerical time by doing away with the manual process of result sorting, but you have also improved confidentiality because results arrive directly in your own intray without third-party intervention.

So the benefits of structured messaging are clear and will apply just as much to discharge summaries and outpatient letters when these too arrive electronically. What new work do they create? The main administrative burden of receiving the results is matching results with patients for whom this is not done automatically. This problem usually arises because of poor addressing by the practice, bad handwriting (guilty m'lud), poor practices at the hospital or, more usually, from a combination of problems at the two ends. So the practice has to have a procedure for manually matching the results with the correct patient. Someone must be identified to do this job, with a deputy to stand in for them when they are away. This is not onerous and amounts to less than 5% of results in my practice. Improved awareness of the import- ance of clear labelling of specimens and request forms at the practice and accurate entry at the trust reduces the number of failed matches, as does use of the new NHS number – so it is useful for something! In the future electronic requesting should solve this problem almost completely and, as an interim, two-dimensional bar coding can automate the process just as effectively.

What happens when I'm away? With paper my secretary just bundles up my results and puts them in my partner's intray. Can you do that with electronic messages? Yup, it's simple, just identify someone (probably the same someone who matches unmatched patients) to forward all Dr B's results to Dr C when they are on holiday. You may want to do this on a daily basis, manually going to Dr B's intray and highlighting and forwarding all results to the covering partner, or automate the system to do it. The problem with the latter is that you have to remember to change it back on the absent doctor's return.

There is the result in your e-intray. It has automatically been date stamped on receipt but where is the action stamp? It will be there, just not imprinted on the result yet. Your system supplier should provide you with some standard options such as 'normal', plus the ability to add free text comments or your own practice's actions. The electronic stamp should have many more options than its rubber equivalent, yet only add those that are relevant to that individual result. In the same way as you might forward the result to another member of the practice for action or filing, you need to be able to do the same thing with paper. Filing is easy. When you have added the result saying 'normal' or 'no action' just click the button that says 'file' and it's filed. Not costing you time and saving your receptionists plenty.

Results that require action by another practice member are a little more complicated. Ideally, what you want is to forward the result to your nurse, for instance, with a note for the patient that says 'please come in for a repeat full blood count in two weeks'. You may or may not want to check that the patient has been notified of this. You want the choice to keep the result in your e-intray until the action has been carried out or be moved completely to the nurse's intray. This requires the ability to leave the result in your intray after filing and for a status for the action to be added. Our system allows actions to be 'outstanding' (not 'marvellous' but 'still to be done'), 'completed', or 'cancelled'. The action in turn may be 'routine' or 'urgent'. These combinations then allow monitoring of results through to completion by the responsible clinician and prioritising of work by the receiver. So that full blood count you sent to the nurse sits in your intray and you see its status change to actioned. Now you know the patient has been notified, you can breathe a sigh of relief and delete the result from your e-intray. The obligatory audit trail shows the full sequence of actions, allowing another layer of security. This ability to manage actions will, for most practices, improve the robustness of their results management and for those that have a results book it will save hours and hours. And when we finally complete the loop with electronic requesting systems, we can be notified when expected results do not arrive in a timely fashion, greatly enhancing reliability of end-to-end messaging.

It is getting the result into the record that really makes the difference; don't be fobbed off with the offer of browsing the trust system. Think of what you can do with the result when it is integrated with the patient record. When Mrs Grundy comes in for the review of her salazopyrin for her rheumatoidarthritis, you can display at the click of a button her white blood count for the last three years or display it graphically to see the effect of medication change and pick up a downward trend to allow tighter monitoring. INRs can be integrated with anticoagulation monitoring programmes, which have been clearly shown to be better than doctor control alone without IT support. Patients who are on lithium for hypomania should have regular lithium blood level checks. They sometimes slip through the net. Well, they did in my practice. Since getting the results of these tests back electronically our clinical system looks for the presence of a lithium test in the last three months whenever we attempt to prescribe lithium. If it does not find one an automatic on-screen reminder pops up advising us to ensure the patient has their lithium levels checked. It does not matter who issues the repeat prescription either – GP, nurse or a non-clinician such as our receptionist. They get the reminder and can therefore make a clinical intervention to improve patient care without needing the clinical experience or expertise. It's not just lithium alone but most chronic diseases where we should regularly monitor blood or urine tests – thyroid disease, patients on diuretics or disease-modifying agents for rheumatoidarthritis, patients with occlusive arterio-vascular disease on statins . . . the list goes on and on, as do the benefits from just having the results on our systems.

Search, research and audit

This is where the computer really excels. It takes me less than five minutes to look at those patients with satisfactory HBA1c levels for diabetes. A real salutary lesson the first time we did it! I can now not only identify those diabetics with poor control to target for more input or agree to accept the poor control, but can also see how we are improving things over time in the practice as a whole. How are you doing at lipid lowering? The new ischaemic heart disease NSF looms large and your PCT will want to know. With the results on board you can see how well things are going *and* demonstrate the enormity of the job still to be done. Even contracting is improved. Do you want to bring in near-patient testing for anticoagulant monitoring? It's usually a damn sight more convenient for patients to come to the surgery and get instant feedback on dosage change. Well, with all laboratory INRs back on our system we were able to show that our patients were getting three times the number of INRs than the papers would tell us to expect. This would have resulted in a gross underestimate of the number of tests and would have left us thousands of pounds out of pocket if we had just accepted the health authority figures we were given and implemented near-patient warfarin monitoring.

Our professional bodies have agreed the standards and content of the information we need for pathology, haematology, microbiology and radiology messaging. The capability to deliver these messages lies within most of the major GP clinical systems suppliers. So why don't we reach up and grab this low-hanging fruit and improve our lives? Well, it's the other end of the link that is often the problem. Does our local pathology laboratory or X-ray department have the capability to squirt out the message containing the right information in the right format over NHSnet or Racal Healthlink? The answer all too often is no. They have to cope with tasks like Read Coding the information accurately and managing the process of sending results electronically, as well as changing their system to add the messaging functionality or getting a middle-ware supplier to add an interface that can do this. At the same time they still have to carry out their everyday work of sending results to GPs, wards and outpatients. The laboratories have only just been notified of the standards they must achieve so many are off to a standing start. A checking service to demonstrate on a trust-by-trust basis that they are putting out high-quality information is only now in the process of being implemented and the funding provided. But it will happen and happen soon. So how do you change from paper to electronic results?

Before you start electronic messaging look closely at what you do with paper. Walk a few reports around the building and make a note of who does what with which, when and why. Then think about what you are likely to do with an electronic results system and how you will manage the receipt of both . . . parallel running. Is it going to require more work during the change over? Probably yes I'm afraid. How will you manage the change? At what point will you sign off the electronic results for patient care and when will you switch off the paper? If you are the first practice of your particular GP system to receive results are you going to require a longer proving period before making the changes? Can you get extra resources from the health authority for the responsibility of being a trailblazer and the extra demands on your time that this involves? What fall back position is there if things go wrong? There will be one but if you ask the laboratory or the health authority and you have the answer it can be very reassuring for your more reluctant partners! Who will end up with the responsibility for matching unmatched patients and other new tasks? What can you do with the time saved by not pulling notes? In our practice when we switched to electronic results for pathology messaging we found that a third of consultations required notes to be pulled to view a pathology report. A third of consultations needed no access to the paper record and a third needed access for radiology reports or hospital letters. So when we switched to pathology messaging for patient care it became a more efficient use of receptionist time to pull just the notes we needed (the last third) for surgeries on an ad-hoc basis. Our receptionists loved it. Pulling and tracking notes is deadly dull. We have trained several receptionists as phlebotomists . . . about one full-time equivalent for a list of 8350 because we no longer pull notes for the majority of surgeries. This has allowed us to increase the use of our practice nurses toward an extended role as nurse practitioners and given the GPs more time for the complex problems. This is a vital safety valve in coping with the burgeoning demand. We expect radiology messaging and discharge and outpatient letters to give us similar additional gains in efficiency.

One of the biggest problems to overcome is familiarity. We recognise a full blood count in an instant and can scan it for abnormalities at a glance. Our eyes recognise the pattern. So when someone comes along and reverses the order of the Hb, WBC and platelet count our eyes stumble and we get frustrated and irritated. So, we should ensure that what we get electronically from the laboratory follows the layout and appearance of the paper as closely as possible. It makes the process of change much easier. Train all the users of the software, from receptionist through nurse to GP. Involve everyone in the change over, as in most practices result management is a group process. It is ever so easy to make assumptions and get things wrong if another key colleague is not there. Getting the doubters involved is vital too. They need an opportunity to express their fears and be heard. If this happens people are much less likely to attempt to sabotage the process.

Trialability is important in helping people to adopt an innovation. It can be had vicariously by a trip to another practice who are established users of electronic messaging. I almost invariably find that practices are happy to share ideas and always come away with something new from just about every different practice I visit. There are also a number of Beacon practices who run sessions on IT and clinical messaging from whose experiences you can learn. Trialability can also be assisted in practice not just from having a demonstration by your system supplier but also by implementing messaging bit by bit. Start with a partner or two viewing and filing the messages, with the whole practice still using paper for patient care. Start with just one message flow, X-ray maybe or pathology. This allows both experience and the reassurance that the technology does what it is supposed to and gives a feel for how the software supports patient management. In particular, how will the practice add comments to the results and manage the filing of those results while at the same time dealing with patient enquiries and patient recall when a result is found to be abnormal? If paper is still being used to manage patients then the electronic processes can be experimented with to see whether the provisional plan for results management does what it is supposed to do. The next step is for the initial GP users to use the reports in parallel with the paper system, which draws in other members of the team: the practice manager to monitor the daily receipt of reports, the receptionist to match unmatched patients and deal with patient enquiries and the practice nurse to deal with patient recall after abnormalities are found.

What is probably becoming clear is that the key to making clinical messaging work is ensuring that the right processes are in place to ensure that electronic results can be used effectively for patient care. This requires a team approach. So, once we have put together a mini team to show that the processes work it can be rolled out to the whole practice. This may take several iterations of process implementation, change and review before finally being rolled out, and minor changes will probably be necessary before everyone is happy.

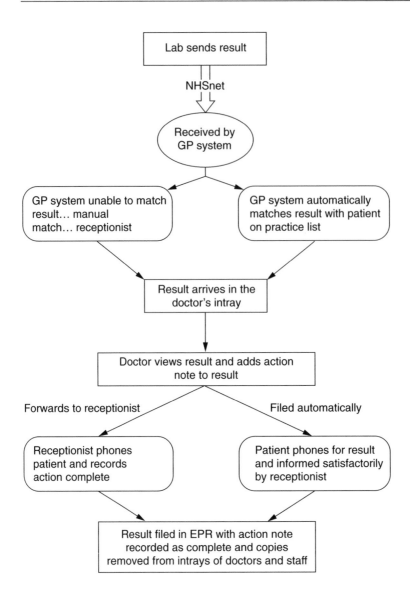

Figure 5.1 Result process flowchart.

6
Getting IT mobile

Even though there has been a considerable shift away from routine home visiting over the last ten years, home visits still form an integral part of the care we offer patients. The care we provide at home is often to our sickest patients and so high-quality information is at least as essential here as it is in a surgery setting. As the swing away from hospital care to home care occurs so community nurses are taking on ever more responsible roles, yet they often do so in what is virtually an information vacuum. How do we provide this information?

The Lloyd George envelope, which was a robust and convenient data storage device for home visits capable of presenting information of multiple types from multiple sources, is being replaced by a computer record that is often none of these. It is a major challenge for primary care informatics to present a complete EPR to those clinicians providing care at home or at the bedside. At the moment there is no perfect replacement that has the characteristics of robustness and compactness whilst being able to store a complete record containing GP notes, letters and investigations. Such solutions are, however, just around the corner, so how do we prepare for them and what do we do in the mean time?

When we look at the needs for information in the surgery one of the first things we find is that we do not have a complete record even there. Pathology messaging places some results in records in some practices but series results such as creatinine clearance or glucose tolerance tests come back manually. Few practices get X-ray and microbiology reports and few scan letters into the EPR. For the vast majority of practices the paper record still stores much of this information and the historical medical record. So before we can provide this at home we have to ensure the surgery-based record is complete. This inevitably means manually entering data from paper format into electronic. Practices need to institute a programme for placing these paper data flows onto the EPR and in the intervening period will need a copy of the paper patient record and the electronic one to take on home visits. In my practice we take the Lloyd George envelope and a printed summary record that contains the last three consultations and all the latest investigations. This is inevitably a compromise in terms of information availability but has the advantage that when admission is required the summary can be sent with a letter to give detailed information to the admitting doctor. So the first step towards having a useful record for home visits is to develop a complete record at the surgery.

When the record is complete at the surgery it is possible with most GP systems to download that information onto a notebook PC that can then be taken by the visiting clinician to the patient's home. This requires knowing which patients are to be visited before leaving our base, which is not always the case. How often do we get calls to see another patient at home when we are already out on our rounds? All too frequently in my experience. So we end up with no patient record except that which resides in our memory. In addition to this, to keep the mobile record and the surgery record synchronised the practice record has to be locked until the updated mobile record is uploaded. This may cause difficulties before weekends and for part-time partners who may not wish to return to the surgery just to upload a record. 'Ruggedised' notebooks that can withstand being dropped are very expensive and cumbersome. Notebooks are also particularly vulnerable to being stolen and there are considerable security implications when the complete patient record is downloaded onto the notebook. The portable record must be password protected for log on and the data on it encrypted for true security.

Ideally, we want to be able to log on to the surgery system from the patient's home, browse the record and log off with no information being downloaded locally. Security then lies with the procedures for logging in to the surgery system, not with the mobile unit. The unit we use has to be capable of displaying the full patient record in a way that can be easily assimilated even in poor lighting conditions. Data entry should also be possible whilst balancing the unit with one hand and entering the information with the other. I don't want any delay in the time it takes to start up as I am already running late and I certainly don't want to have to plug it in to a local power supply or the patient's telephone. This really rules out anything other than a mini-laptop or a hand-held device. The average laptop is far too heavy to hold in one hand and a WAP phone screen of less than two inches square is really far too small to present the quantity and layout of information we need for patient care. My hand-held device must also be capable of running software that can display my clinical system and allow me to enter information easily and quickly. Not a lot to ask is it? I would also like it to have other uses such as diary and office functions that are compatible and can synchronise with my PC. So my shortlist might include products from:

- Psion, Series 5, Revo (hand-held) or Series 7 (mini-notebook)
  http://www.psion.com

- Nokia communicator integral phone and PDA
  http://www.nokia.com

- Palm Pilot, Vx (palm-top)
  http://www.palm.com

- Casio, Cassiopeia (palm-top)
  http://www.casio.com

- Hewlett Packard, Jornada and pocket PC
  http://www.hewlettpackard.com

- Sony, Clie (palm-top) Viaio PCG–C1XS – not instant start up but it is a real Windows notebook
  http://www.sony.com

- Hitachi, the one to watch? HPW 630EPR
  http://www.hitachi.com

New devices are coming on to the market nearly every day so I would use my checklist (*see* Box 6.1) to see which is most likely to suit me! Most of these devices require a mobile phone to communicate with the surgery and if you have a Windows-based system, downloading screens over a mobile is going to seem interminably slow with current GSM transmission rates.

Box 6.1 Portable requirements checklist

- Lightweight
- Robust
- Compact
- Rechargeable/standard batteries
- Screen of at least half VGA 320*640
- Integral modem/radio link to GSM phone
- Touch sensitive screen/integral keyboard
- Instant start up
- Backlit display (for poor ambient light)
- Compatible client software

Even when you have the full record on the system, how are you going to issue the prescription without a portable printer? No one is going to hump around a portable printer to issue prescriptions, so the logical fudge is to continue to issue them by hand or print them off at the surgery and send them to the chemist. Roll on 2004 and electronic prescription exchange with pharmacies.

Though slow, this dial up method of connecting a PDA (personal digital assistant) over a mobile phone connection is being used in a pilot in Avon to give community nurses access to their patient-based clinical records. It seems to significantly improve job satisfaction, adds to the EPR and benefits patient care. It has to be the way to go, doesn't it?

7
Painless prescriptions and pen-less prescribing

The use of computers for prescribing was one of the earliest steps towards automation in general practice and also one of the most potent motivators for the adoption of computerisation. Hours spent recording repeat prescriptions in triplicate, writing them, updating reminder cards and entering the issue in the patient's Lloyd George or A4 record, were liberated. Now the vast majority of GPs perform all these functions with just a couple of keystrokes or delegate virtually the whole repeat prescription process to a member of the administration team. This leaves the doctor with the simple duty of authorising the prescription with their signature. How come even this seems arduous? The answer is not hard to find. Rising demand, new treatments and the shift of chronic disease management into primary care have all conspired to increase the number of prescriptions issued, as well as the complexity of the medications prescribed. Computers have become an essential tool for managing this intricate environment and have the potential to do more still. This chapter will explore what they can do and what they will be expected to do.

One of the key mechanisms we have for the management of illness is the issue of a medication to the sufferer. Potent new treatments come on to the market almost every day with potent new side-effects, contraindications and interactions.

Investigations are used for monitoring effect and response to treatment in the individual and the penalty for error in this ever more litigious society gets ever more severe. At the same time government and health authorities of every kind are placing pressure on the prescriber to issue fewer and more cost-effective prescriptions. Can the computer save us from all these conflicting demands? Certainly computers can make the process of issuing prescriptions faster and reduce the errors arising from the apocryphal medical dysgraphia. Few would contest that. Most of us have experienced this first hand in our practices through the simple first step of entering all repeat prescriptions on the computer.

Acute prescribing by computer is the next step for most practices on the road to the EPR. It's crazy not to, isn't it? Many prescriptions are only acute prescriptions the first time they are issued. You see the hypertensive patient after the usual work-up and start them on an ACE inhibitor and issue a four-week script. Back they come as planned with a BP down to 120/70. Great. You issue a repeat and review three months later. You have just put them on a repeat of the same medication that you issued acutely last month. It makes sense to use the computer for the initial issue, does it not? And, of course, being the practical people we are, that is what most of us now do and in a single step the computer is being used during the consultation.

The logic continues. We are now using the clinical system for all of our prescribing, acute and chronic. So if we are entering all medication on the computer, why don't we use the system as an aide-mémoire? It does not take much programming to create a few rules to look for a record of drug allergies in the patient record, and we need never again worry about inducing an anaphylactic reaction that may kill the patient and land us in court. Of course, that requires us to enter all known drug allergies on the computer. We can do our best to enter the allergies and so reduce the risk for our patients and ourselves even if we never reach the stage of perfection! If we can do it for allergies then we can do it for interactions, can't we? That should be even easier because interactions are not patient-specific. We just have to get someone to plug away at the computer entering all the interaction data into the database and create a rule that says, 'display a screen message saying BEWARE if the GP should attempt to issue drug A at the same time as drug B'. So that is what our GP system suppliers have done.

Our patients are, of course, individuals. We all know that contraindications may be absolute or relative and we know our patients as those individuals. We, the GP, weigh up the risks of prescribing or not and evaluate one medication against an alternative in each unique human being in each unique situation. Provided, that is, we have the necessary knowledge or have access to it. New drugs and failing memories, human ones that is, mean that access to information is vital and that is what computers can do very well. They can give access to information when and where it is required to the level of detail that is required. So here is the next logical step: the BNF on-line and e-MIMS. The pharmaceutical compendium is at our fingertips or mouse click and if one or the other is not integrated into your clinical system in some way, it should be.

We know all our patients' individual histories and circumstances and recollect and weigh up all their illnesses when we prescribe, don't we? Well, I don't I'm afraid. I try to, but occasionally some of the information escapes me. I have, I can confess, prescribed ibuprofen to someone with a past history of peptic ulcer that I had not noted. No harm came to them but who knows what the consequences might be the next time this happens. If I have noted the key diagnosis of peptic ulceration in the computer (a Read-coded entry of course!) the computer can give me a good talking to if I attempt to prescribe the wrong medication. All it takes is a few more rules in the software and me to build up a comprehensive morbidity register, and I will not prescribe a medication with individual contraindications for a patient again. The patient is safer from harm and we are safer from litigation, good news all around.

But I want my patients to have more than safety; I want them to have the best possible care and that often means the best possible medication. In the hypertensive West Indian diabetic with mild renal impairment I saw this morning, let's call him Thomas Good, what is the most appropriate first-line treatment for his blood pressure? What does the evidence say? Computer software can help. All it needs is a few more rules and some patient information to work on and access to a cornucopia of evidence for one effective treatment distilled by the great and the good. It needs me to enter coded information for ethnicity, diabetes, hypertension, renal impairment and gender into the patient record. In a millisecond the computer can give me a list of preferred treatments tailored to this individual and explain why, so that I have a better idea about what to choose next time. Of course, most of the time common things occur commonly and I will not usually need this support but it's great to have on hand when you do. This sort of decision support is a brilliant tool for the new registrar or for giving a safe if restricted choice of treatments to the new nurse prescriber. The NHS has commissioned just such a tool that is compatible with the major GP systems. It's called Prodigy, a derivative of a Dutch concept that made for significantly more cost-effective prescribing. The cost saving was not nearly so marked in the UK system, probably because most GPs in the trial were already doing a pretty good job as cost-effective prescribers. Small savings were made and it is now available for all of us to use. Of particular benefit is the production of patient advice, in addition to the prescription, as an outcome of the decision support. It makes the process faster as well as potentially more effective.

Money saving in prescribing is unfortunately a driving force that often conflicts with good prescribing. If I suffer a penalty for expensive prescribing it is inevitable that I will tend to prescribe more cheaply and my values system will justify it. I am only human! This is not what I want to do. So any tool that helps me prescribe cost effectively and well, I welcome. So I generally welcome Prodigy as I do the fact that my computer can automatically suggest a generic substitute if I try and prescribe a branded one. They are usually cheaper and usually an appropriate choice. Generic medications are not however always the cheapest choice. We are increasingly seeing cheaper branded alternatives for many generics and it requires an encyclopaedic brain to stay up to date, not only with the latest drugs but also with the changes in their prices. Not surprisingly software is available that can offer us the choice of the least expensive alternative to the medication we have selected, irrespective of whether it is generic or branded. We can decide to override the offer or select the recommended product as we wish. One such product, Scriptswitch, does all this at the point of prescription issue and so can work with decision support tools such as Prodigy. Tools that help us stay within budget help keep the pressure off prescribing according to cost rather than clinical need.

You remember Thomas Good, my patient with diabetes, hypertension and mild renal impairment and how decision-support tools can offer care tailored to his individual condition? Well, it requires all those Read Codes to be recorded in the notes to make the appropriate decisions. So it is essential for us to use coded entries for conditions that may affect prescribing, renal and hepatic impairment being two of the most important. These should be de rigueur in any practice morbidity database. However, now that we are getting pathology results back in coded format and integrated with the patient's electronic record, there is an opportunity to put in place a safety net. Say we have performed a blood test for creatinine and electrolytes during Thomas's hypertensive work up. The result of the creatinine comes back at 120 mmol/l. I try to prescribe an ACE inhibitor. Rules in my computer system look for both a Read Code for mild renal impairment and a code for blood creatinine level with a value greater than 100 mmol/l. When I attempt to prescribe an ACE inhibitor it finds a creatinine of 120 mmol/l, 'beware' pops up and I am reminded of the risk of continuing with this medication. Getting pathology results back electronically automatically populates our GP systems with information that, provided the right rules are present to make use of the information, can improve the safety of our prescribing. We have not had to enter a thing by hand in the process! This is the added value of having a complete EPR, so don't diss it!!

Our clinical systems have helped us produce the most specific and cost-effective prescription for our patients but we still have to print it out and hand it to the patient to take to the pharmacist. When the pharmacist gets it they have to send it to the Prescription Pricing Authority (PPA). In darkened rooms in Leeds rows of grim figures with heads bowed over piles of dog-eared slips of green paper tap data into computers that duplicate the information that our computers have printed out. They are grim because they can see redundancy looming as their role as middlemen becomes unnecessary. Sorry people but you really could be doing something more productive. By 2008 or even earlier the NHS Plan tells us that transfer of prescription data between GPs, pharmacies and the PPA will take place electronically for the majority of us. So there we have it. A deadline for literally hundreds of data-entry clerks when their jobs will go and a deadline for us when we must be routinely sending prescriptions electronically to our local pharmacies. This will start to be piloted in three areas by June 2001. This means that practices that are not using a clinical computer system for acute and repeat prescribing need to start doing so now! For the majority of GPs who already do this there is little to do but sit back and wait for our system suppliers and the NHSIA to produce software that will do the job safely. The electronically-produced prescriptions will have digital signatures that carry the same legal force as prescriptions signed in writing. So repeat prescribing will become pen-less as well as painless!!

E-pharmacy also deserves a mention as it is flagged in the NHS Plan for a higher profile. The Government's view is that there is no reason why medicines should not be sold or dispensed electronically, and nothing to preclude distance sale and supply like mail order or home delivery. They will be actively looking at ways to facilitate this with NHS prescriptions. The short-term expectation is for electronic consultations with pharmacists with the prescription being delivered manually. Electronic consultations with pharmacists, eh? What does that herald for GPs whose business is the consultation? I think we have been warned!

Many local pharmacists believe that there is a serious threat from warehouse pharmacies delivering medications to the door. We too should probably be concerned as the personal knowledge of practices and patients by neighbourhood pharmacies helps ensure detection of errors in prescribing and the delivery of personal advice to our patients. Loss of this is likely to be an automatic consequence of the automation of prescription dispensing, which itself is probably inevitable. How we safeguard the security that our local chemist services often provide will no doubt sorely test us all.

If we look towards the middle of the first decade of the new millennium and prescribing in primary care we might see consulting rooms without printers, prescriptions authorised by the touch of a mouse pointer and drugs delivered to patients' homes by a national courier service, drugs that have been picked off shelves in a warehouse by a mechanical hand. Instruction labels will be attached to the packet and passed on conveyor belt under the gaze of a production-line pharmacist who checks the issue against the computer screen before the carrier collects it for the journey to the patient, who may be hundreds of miles away! The revolution in prescribing and dispensing will be one of the major changes brought about by the computerisation of primary care. How could it not be? It is such a large part of what we do. We need to grasp this challenge and make sure that its implementation works for our patients, our practice and our profession.

8
Scanning

How can we ever reach a state of paperlessness when every day over the reception desk, in the post and on faxes that fade and make the illegible invisible, paper pours into the surgery? The answer is simple – scan it. Yet although the answer is simple, the process is not. I don't mean the actual process of scanning, putting a piece of paper into a machine much like a photocopier and pressing a button. That's easy enough. No, the process by which we manage that electronic image once it is in the computer and how we make it part of a useful electronic record. There's no point in just getting rid of the paper. Did I really say that? I did and I'm right, there really *is* no benefit from getting rid of paper if we cannot use the electronic copy in a way that is at least as effective as the original in running our practices and caring for our patients. So, in this chapter the perils and benefits of scanning will be explored so that in your practice the road to the electronic record ends up with a complete record, comprising the knowledge from all the pieces of paper that arrive.

Scanning in practice?

So start at the beginning. What is scanning? Scanning is the process of taking a document and copying it into an electronic format. Ink on paper becomes an electronic image of the original, a facsimile in fact. A fax machine does just this before it converts the image into pulses and squirts it down the wire. A scanner is like a truncated fax but instead of being linked to BT or Cable and Wireless, it has a wire that plugs into the back of a PC and the image is sent to a programme that allows you to display the image on screen. Every new scanner comes with software that can do this, as without it you would just have bought a box with a glass lid and a light behind it. Not a lot of use in the paperless surgery, I'm afraid.

To scan something you put the paper onto the scanner or into its feeder mechanism, press a button, either on the scanner or on the software, and, after a few buzzes and whirrs, the image appears on screen. This document image can then simply be stored on your computer – but if it is about a patient, it needs to be linked in some way to the patient record to which it refers, more of which later. Where we receive printed text documents, however, the technology allows us to do something smarter than making an electronic photograph of the original. Special software known as OCR (optical character recognition software because it recognises optical characters, or recognises characters optically) looks at the electronic image that you have just scanned in and says that e-dots in that shape represent the letter T, for example. It then stores this as the computer code for a letter, rather than the information for lots of e-dots, which occupies much less of the computer's memory. It then proceeds to the next discrete set of e-dots and recognises an H and stores this, then an R and stores this. Now it gets clever, THR then a space tells the software that this should be a word. It then compares it with its dictionary but like your temporary non-medical secretary who has never come across THR before, brings this misspelling to your attention by flashing . . . doesn't your secretary do that? . . . or by underlining or highlighting it in red to bring it to your notice. You then look at it and tell the computer it is ignorant and should in future recognise the abbreviation for total hip replacement by adding it to the dictionary. Next time it comes across THR it will accept it. It then goes through the whole letter in this way converting images into digitally stored codes for the characters that make up words. Why do I care? Is it because the OCRd text occupies 1/1000 of the memory? No. Is it because the spelling has been checked? No. It *is* because the characters are stored as computer code, not e-dots, and these can then be stored as meaningful text (assuming the original was meaningful!) in any compatible word processing programme, such as that in your clinical system for instance, as part of the EPR. Not only that, because these converted dots now carry meaning, other clever programmes can search them and help you find and extract important clinical information. It becomes simple to move this information between programmes, into e-mail perhaps or into a new referral letter. The information is now portable. It can even be integrated into your clinical system and form part of the patient's electronic health record. You can scan in all your letters and shred the original. No filing, marvellous, letters wherever you need them whenever you need them, marvellous. You are paperless overnight, marvellous. Quick, which scanner should we buy? Hang on a moment though. There are problems too, so read on.

Pitfalls

You understand the process of scanning; dots on paper are converted into meaningful information by clever software. Well, just as the inexperienced secretary can change meaning by guessing so can this not-so-clever software. A dot on a piece of paper may be a full stop or a decimal point or a piece of dirt, and the clever software tries to guess which. If it is dirt, it should ignore it. If it is the decimal point in a drug dosage that is going to be used as a reference to change a patient's medication, it may be quite literally vital. Even if really clever software (I don't think such a thing exists yet) could understand drug dosage values in the middle of text, it cannot account for varying ages or clinical situations. Missing a decimal point because the computer thought it was dirt could easily result in a patient receiving ten times the intended dose of medication. It would require careful scrutiny by a clinician to detect such computer-generated changes, a clinician who will need to refer to the original. You cannot do this if you have shredded it. A well-trained scanning clerk would frequently be able to identify changes in the meaning of text when the software gets it wrong and even correct the grammar in the original, but to be responsible for checking doses and values of results where accurate numbers are crucial is too much to expect.

You want to start scanning and OCRing incoming patient letters because you want this information whenever you need it and wherever you are in the practice. You want to get rid of all that mind-numbing filing of letters and pulling of notes so your receptionists can use their time for something more productive. Can scanning save you time? Well, there are certainly huge timesavings for the doctors and nurses in being able to view letters at the touch of a button, but for scanning clerks who were probably receptionists in a former existence it is not necessarily the case. Loading sheets of paper takes time, scanning the image takes time, using OCR software takes time and checking for errors and moving the text into your clinical system all take time. When you implement scanning solutions in your practice great care needs to be taken to ensure that these processes are done as time efficiently as possible.

Box 8.1 Hints for fast scanning and OCR

- Buy a fast PC on which to run the software (600MHz PIII is ideal) with lots (128MB) of memory.

- Buy a fast scanner, look at both the time to scan (some take a while to warm up) and the time per scan.

- Get a scanner with a SCSI interface (connection) to the computer. Parallel port and USB scanners transmit the information to the computer more slowly.

- Get a sheet-fed scanner to allow batch scanning.

- Don't scan at high resolution (more than 300 dots per inch) for optical character recognition. It is slower, uses more memory and picks up more background artefacts that it tries to convert into text.

- Scan text documents in black and white *not* colour.

- Buy the best possible OCR software available.

- Become familiar with your OCR software: some software learns to improve its text recognition with use, make sure this facility is switched on.

- Batch scan documents with different typefaces together, particularly if a dot matrix printer has produced them. You can vastly improve recognition if the software is told that it is about to receive scanned dot matrix text or a particular font.

- Visit a practice that uses scanning and learn from their successes and mistakes.

- Automate repetitive keystrokes with macros, a single key or key combination that has the action of multiple keystrokes, e.g. a single keystroke selects the OCR text, copies it to the computer's clipboard and pastes it into the clinical systems wordprocessor. If you cannot create a macro, get someone to set up the system to do this for you. It's worth every penny!

Kit

OK, so now which scanner or software should we buy? You know the features your scanner needs for OCR work because they are listed in Box 8.1 and a scanner that can do all of this will set you back about £300 including VAT for a Hewlett Packard 6300c. This can scan at resolutions of up to 1200 dots per inch, well above what you need for OCR work, but a higher resolution might be useful for transferring images into your practice leaflet or newsletter using desktop publishing software. Other names to look out for are Epson and Fujitsu. The latter has recently produced a scanner, the 3091DC, that can process 15 pages per minute, three times as many as the Hewlett Packard, but it has a maximum resolution of only 600 dpi, half that of the Hewlett Packard but more than enough for most normal practice uses. If you are a larger practice the £550 price tag may well be worth it for the speed. Its

---

Box 8.2 Uses of scanning

- Converting printed letters to text for integration in the EPR.
- Copying handwritten reports for attachment to the EPR.
- Storing images, e.g. ECGs can be scanned as black-and-white images and attached to the patient record.
- For computerised fax systems . . . very useful if lots of people will be sent the same fax.
- Copying and storing information from PCG/health authority or Department of Health in an electronic format.
- Copying pictures for inclusion in practice documents and newsletters.
- Creating an electronic library of reference articles scanned from magazines.*

*Bear in mind copyright restrictions

maximum daily page rate is 250, which should be plenty for practices of eight or even ten whole-time partners.

As your reliance on scanning increases so does your dependence on the process so having a backup scanner may be useful; basic scanners can be purchased for well under £100. The hardware changes all the time so be on the lookout for hardware that does the job you need it to do. Not only should it be fast, it should be compact, have a sheet feeder and be quiet in operation. This last factor is tremendously important in a small office environment. A noisy scanner or computer can alienate a lot of people so when looking for a new scanner, listen for one too. One more thing to consider is whether you will be scanning two-sided documents. If you expect a lot of these then go for a duplex scanner, which scans both sides of the page automatically.

That's the hardware, what about the software? Well, as you know (and I know you know because I told you just now) the more accurate the software the better. As each new version leapfrogs the competition you may be changing your software every year or 18 months but as upgrades tend to be inexpensive this is often well worth doing. The two big kids on the block in OCR terms are Text Bridge and Omnipage and these two arch rivals have pushed the development cycle and accuracy ever faster. Now, however, the takeover of the latter by Xerox means that the pressure may be off these two for the time being, although the convergence of the technology behind these products may mean further improvements in accuracy. They still exist in their separate identities with minor differences in function but there is probably not a lot to choose between them. Subtleties such as the ability to scan into forms or to convert text directly into HTML may be the sort of difference that helps you choose one over the other. The ability to convert to HTML means that you can take a document and instantly convert it to a web page that can be used on the practice Intranet or on your website. The trick here is for the software to preserve the appearance of the original it came from. My experience is that this still leaves a lot to be desired as a one-click process, but is a useful step in converting documents for publishing on the Web, even though most will need polishing in an HTML editor of some sort (Frontpage, Dreamweaver or the like).

There is probably one other product you should think about when considering scanning in your practice. That is Adobe Acrobat, currently in its fourth iteration. You may know the name as it is a de-facto standard for communicating documents whilst retaining their original appearance. Every PC user needs the Adobe Acrobat reader as many NHS documents are published in this format. The reader is free. Download it from the Web or get a copy from your health authority – it's an essential if you don't have it already. The reader does not help you with scanning but Acrobat 4, which allows you to produce documents in what's known as PDF (portable document format) direct from your scanner, does. This means that anyone with the free reader can see your document as it was intended to be seen. You can even sign your document and prevent it from being changed or edited in any way. Using Acrobat you can scan a document and it is effectively a facsimile of the original so that the risks from errors occurring when you use OCR software are not there. You can scan a letter into Adobe PDF and attach it to the patient's record. If you view it later it is as if you see a copy of the original. It still takes up much more space than the OCRd text and cannot be fully integrated into a text-based GP system. But for many using a combination of OCR and PDF (Adobe) it is the way to manage letters for inclusion in the EPR. It's an effective copywriting tool if you need it too. It supports images and text in one document and compresses them so they take up less hard disk space and if you are heavily involved in producing documents for teaching or research, your PCG or LMC or just plan to have a comprehensive practice library on your Intranet, you may well get a lot of value from buying Adobe Acrobat, even if you do not plan to use it for a belt and braces clinical letter management process. But . . . it's going to cost you around £350.

It may seem that with electronic messaging and clinical e-mail around the corner the bulk of the incoming data will be in electronic format and therefore the need to scan documents will be redundant even before you have trained your staff to do it. Unfortunately, receiving all our NHS clinical information in electronic format is still a long way off. If we are to rely on an EPR it *must* be complete. Unrecognised missing patient information puts our patients at risk. So, until all NHS organisations are able to send information to one another we must be able to integrate documents into our records. Even if every part of the NHS gets its act together we will still receive documents from solicitors, employers and even handwritten notes on the backs of envelopes from patients, all of which need to be part of the EPR. Yup, scanning is unfortunately going to be with us for a long time yet and achieving a paperless practice is not possible without it for the foreseeable future, so it is probably worth becoming familiar with it now. It is immensely useful.

9
The Internet, the Web and the practice

The World Wide Web is the software standard from CERN, which provides a simple and standard way to find and view documents on the Internet. The Internet is the computer, data, telecommunications links and software that allow the transmission of data between connected computers throughout the world.

Right, so now we know . . . onto the next chapter! Well, the Internet is changing so fast maybe that is all we need to know about its history; as soon as anything is written about the Internet it's out of date. More facts might be useful I suppose. More than 11 million people in the States shop online for health products (Cyber Practice Health Dialogue Study if you want to know the source), and 55 million are predicted to follow suit by 2005. They use the Internet for information about disease 46%, treatment 36%, 28% for wellness, whatever that Americanism means (Jupiter 2000). The market is still immature in the UK in terms of market research and data and most of what we know comes from the USA, so I suppose Americanisms are reasonable. What we do know is that health sites are the most commonly visited after pornography . . . no . . . not that we look up the diseases that the porno stars have contracted after viewing the sex sites. No, health is the second most popular topic on the Internet. What is popular is what is there. What is there, available on the Internet, has largely arisen out of academia putting research outcomes on the Web or from a desire for profit by commercial organisations. In the UK more than 30% of people have daily access to the Internet. Eighty per cent of GPs have access compared with more than 90% of American physicians, according to a study by the Royal Society of Medicine. We are following the US model but have a unique opportunity to change how people in the UK use Internet health information because of the way the NHS is organised and delivers healthcare. NHS Direct Online is already showing that. Online diagnoses, prescriptions and even consultations may be the way we are going but they are still a few years away. The Internet and primary care in the UK is virtually a blank page and I would urge you to start filling it.

So that's what the public feels about health on the Net. What can it do for the practice? Well just as we are ordinary consumers of healthcare as well as providers, we are ordinary users of the Internet. I find it brilliant for things like finding train times (http://www.railtrack.com) and travel information. In fact, as I type this in the gentle evening sun overlooking an olive grove in Tuscany and muse on the fact that seven days ago in a rain-sodden Bristol I bought six return flights to Italy for £360 all in and booked an overnight hotel in Pisa online in less than 20 minutes on the Net, I dare anyone to tell me that the Internet is not a wonderful thing! Sante. More mundane, but useful, is to use it for purchasing practice consumables; stationery, ink refills and computer products can all be bought at substantial discounts. Though many of us are still anxious when giving our credit card details over the Internet, it is probably more secure than when your card itself disappears out of sight for 10 minutes at a restaurant. If you find the padlock symbol on the bottom right of your Internet Explorer web browser, you have an encrypted connection for your transaction and even if intercepted the credit card details would be jumbled up and mean nothing to a cybercriminal.

This type of use is not only easy and potentially money saving, it also helps breed familiarity and confidence in using the Net and can only help as practices start to order vaccines and medical goods over the Net. Now if you are happy with the phone for ordering that's fine, but buying on the Web means that you can compare the latest prices. Online software can automatically calculate and display discounts accurately, and order-tracking software can keep you appraised of where in the supply chain your purchase is, from order to dispatch and even to estimated time of delivery. This is a boon for dispensing practices and those ordering lots of esoteric vaccines for their travel clinics, where good stock control can mean both substantial savings and happy patients; it's nigh on impossible, or at least impossibly time consuming, using conventional communication media.

Most doctors start using the Internet in clinical areas, to find articles and clinical information. Familiarity with sources such as Medline and OMNI, which give access to digests of medical references and papers online, are quite rightly often higher on the agenda than e-commerce. These are usually accessed through a third party such as the BMA or the Royal College of General Practitioners online sites, but can really help to keep the practice up to date and not bamboozled when the Thought Police use 'evidence-based care' to mean the least expensive treatment justified by carefully selected 'evidence'!

Being confident in the quality of health information is a significant problem for all of us, doctors and patients alike, who use the Internet. There are a number of organisations that put a stamp of legitimacy on sites. There are the Consumers Association's 'Which' marked sites, which conform to high standards of general information, and HON, the Health On the Net foundation, for health sites whose function is to promote good standards in health information on the Web. Sites are vetted and are allowed to display the Which or HON symbol only if they fulfil certain require-ments. It's really pretty obvious stuff but is all too frequently omitted from some quite authoritative sites. What would you want to know about medical information? Who wrote the information, certainly, when it was updated and you would likely want to see a list of references for background information. Does the author have any financial sponsors or is he selling a product? These things might alter the reader's perception of the information's independence and therefore its objectivity. Look for the HON code in the message but you will still need your critical reading skills for Web publications just as you do for paper-based ones. There are many useful medical sites for GPs on the Web and a list appears at http://www.healthcentral.co.uk/links/gp – dip your toe in the surf!

The BMA and RCGP publish sites with both public and members pages that have lots of useful information and reference pages. Often it is the sort of thing you hardly ever need but when you do you cannot lay your hands on it. Hit the BMA site, log in and do a quick search and there it is, guidelines on X, Y and Z or the relevant statutory instrument. It has taken you moments through your NHSnet connection, at no cost and it's on someone else's filing system to which they have given you the keys. Thanks guys. This is where the Internet excels. It gives us access to virtually unlimited information of every kind in just seconds, provided of course we know where to look. That brings up the subject of searches but we will come back to those in a minute. Let's stay with the concept of someone else maintaining and managing documents for us on the Internet. If they are the original producer or owner of the information, why shouldn't they manage it? Up until now the main reason for us to store copies locally is the cost of accessing the information when we need it, costs in both cash and time. Paying for AOL or CompuServe, paying for usage and paying for phone calls meant that when there was a document we were likely to need more than once, it was most effective to download it onto our own PC. But now all that has changed. How? Well, because of NHSnet and Project Connect (don't ya just lurve those virile names that issue forth from the NHS Executive in a never-ending stream . . . Project Connect . . . to link every GP to NHSnet from their desktop by the end of 2000). The new virile epaulet is needed because the *Information for Health* target of connecting every practice by December 1999 was never achievable, so missing the target had to be dressed in new clothes. Instead of every practice we now have every GP and a target that has slipped again to end of fiscal year 2000. Now I'm not knocking it. Connecting every GP makes a lot more sense, as does a realistic timescale. At least then the possibility of an e-mail revolution in primary care can become a reality. Of course, it should really be every clinician in the NHS, Operation Health Storm perhaps? I digress. All GPs connect from their desktops to NHSnet by ISDN line. No cost for connection, no cost for calls and no cost for kit it seems.

We are talking a new paradigm here (God! It's contagious!!). GPs will have a free pipeline into the NHSnet and the Internet. This is going to change the way we use the Internet before most of us have even started using it. What is this bloke on about, I can almost feel you thinking. Well, the bloke is on about this: fast access to unlimited documents when we want them, links to their progenitors, someone else to store, index, update and publish information in multiple different formats and provide us with sophisticated tools to search them. So, this bloke asks himself, why do I need the same stuff cluttering up my hard disk? The answer I give myself is a simple 'I don't'. Let someone else do all the hard work; all I need to do is maintain my links in a structured way locally. So, when I click on a link I go directly to the document, even if it's held in Connecticut. All I am saying is that we abandon the NHS prerequisite of whenever you need a wheel build your own, and instead say 'OK. It's circular, has spokes and rolls. It does what I want. Thanks for letting me use it!'.

What links do I want?

It may be useful for you to maintain your own list of practice favourites, which can easily be added to Bookmarks (Netscape Navigator) or Favourites (Internet Explorer). Just set up a practice section with subfolders for:

- Government
- NHSIA
- HA
- PCT
- Clinical
- Professional
- Patient resources.

These are examples of high-level folders; each in turn can have subfolders much like Windows Explorer.

I know many people like to have information on their own systems but isn't it better for the BMA for instance to manage their information and the Department of Health its own, without us having to do it? Well, if you think your wheel is going to be rounder and create less drag than theirs, build it! There is information that most of us will want to have on our own machines, local in-house information or that which is shared between a couple of practices, or for organisations that don't have a Web presence. If that organisation is of any size remind it of Darwin's principles and the need to stay fit for purpose. If your trainers' or young principals' group or journal club doesn't have a site, grab your PCT and get them to manage the documents, Website and e-mail list, which allows newsletters and the like to be circulated to all members at the click of just one button. It'll give them something to do with all those IT staff!

There are things that are clearly in-house and obviously should remain so. Included amongst these will be things that are so precious or so frequently used that you would be devastated if you lost them or could not work without them. Personal information, confidential stuff and those things that there would be no purpose in sharing with others outside of the practice, such as accounts and payroll information.

Searching the Web

Most people who use the Web will rapidly discover a vast source of information from which it is often difficult to pick what is relevant. This is no less true for medical resources than it is for general Internet information. First you need to know what you are looking for. Not just approximately but exactly what you are searching for. Most search engines need you to enter 'keywords' that you think the page with the correct information might contain. If your keywords are too vague, you will be overwhelmed by potential information sources. If you search for GP Websites on AltaVista you will find you get 101 578 734 results, some of which are for global positioning systems, which is not really what you want! If your searches are too narrow or too specialised, you may find you get nothing at all.

In principle, using a Web search engine is very simple . . . type in a 'keyword' (one that you would expect to find on the page of information that you are looking for), hit the search button, and back come the URLs of webpages containing the information you are looking for, usually with a brief description or the first few words from the page. In practice, you often need to refine your search very carefully otherwise you will be swamped by many thousands of possible pages. Fortunately, many search engines allow you to define your search accurately using Boolean operators and wildcard characters. The way that these are used often vary slightly from one search engine to another, but what follows generally applies (Box 9.1).

Box 9.1 Search engine tips

AND: 'gp AND websites' will only find those pages which contain **both** of those words.

NOT: 'gp NOT websites' will find the pages that contain the word 'gp' but which **do not** contain the word 'websites'.

Some search engines use plus (+) and minus (-) signs in front of the search words instead of AND and NOT.

OR: 'gp OR websites' will find pages which contain **either** of the two words.

NEAR: 'gp NEAR websites' will find pages which only contain those two words close to each other. This facility is only found on a few search engines.

Wild card characters: Usually the asterisk. 'web*' will find pages with any words beginning with 'web', whilst 'websites*' will find 'websitess' as well as 'websites'.

Double-quotation marks: Enclosing two or more words with "double-quotation marks" will normally cause them to be treated as a phrase, rather than separate words. This applies to nearly all search engines.

Capital letters: Entering your search words in capital letters will **only** find references in capitals. Lower case search words will find both upper and lower case entries. So 'GP' would only find pages with 'GP', but 'gp' would find 'gp', 'GP' or 'gP'. This convention also applies to most search engines.

Intranets

An Intranet is a local network that is separate from or cannot be accessed from the Internet, usually protected by a firewall that keeps it secure. It does, however, utilise Internet browser technology. This means that you can publish practice documents as Webpages, link with hyperlinks and even utilise Internet-type search facilities. This is a great way to manage practice information as once you and your staff know how to surf the Web, using the Intranet is a natural way of working. This has been recognised by the NHS Executive and they have produced an Intranet package called Digerati based around the Microsoft database Access, which can cope with the needs of large practices, PCTs and even trusts. If you have Access it can be virtually free to set up. Most practices will, however, need technical support to implement it, which most will not have in-house. PCTs may in the future offer support in setting up and maintaining Digerati and there are now a number of companies who offer this.

Back to the Intranet. You need a PC to function as your webserver, which provides the pages with links to other documents on your network. This might be any PC on your network, the practice clinical server or a machine dedicated to this purpose. The latter is probably best and if this is all it is required to do you can probably get away with recycling an old machine. Don't forget that it will be used as the file system for lots of your important practice documents, so it will need back-up facilities. Use the back-up in just the same manner as your clinical system. You use the Web design software to produce webpages that link to files on your system and, provided your PCs all have the viewer software or the full program and a web browser such as Internet Explorer, they can simply surf to any of the linked documents and view them. With so much information that can potentially be stored this way, careful thought needs to be given to your file structure to ensure time is not wasted looking for documents. If you use Microsoft Office software, the viewer software for Word and Excel is free and cannot run viruses, so you don't have to go to the expense of installing the full software on every PC in your network. Adobe Acrobat is another excellent tool (I repeat myself because I don't want you to miss out!) as it stores text and images in one document as well as compressing files so they take up less space. The viewer is free and is a universally recognised medium so should not prove a problem if you subsequently need to forward such documents out of the practice! To produce Webpages, however, you will need to learn a bit about HTML, the language of the Internet, but it is not too hard to learn and much of the basic software to set up Webpages is available free, e.g. FrontPage Express.

The practice on the Web

More than 50% of businesses have websites yet only around 400 practices, according to latest Government figures, have a Web presence. That is less than 5% of all practices in the UK. Why the difference? I can only assume that there is little perceived commercial benefit from producing a website for GPs. As usual for general practice however, where there is no carrot we find a stick to encourage us forward. In September 2000, the Government issued advice that all NHS organisations should provide information for publication on the Web and on links to their sites. http://www.doh.gov.uk/nhsexipu/whatnew/eguide.html. Paragraph 6.2 of which states:

The first action for all NHS organisations is to ensure they have a Web editor and for health authorities in particular to ensure they have the capacity and resources to co-ordinate and edit the core information.

So, who is going to be the Web Czar in your practice?

There are good reasons for a practice going to the trouble of developing their own website, beyond the fact that patients expect it. It gives patients instant access to practice information without having to queue at reception or hang on waiting for the phone to be answered. As this demand is increasing exponentially and cannot usually be met by existing personnel and resources, we need every tool that can help us. Not only that, the Internet can deliver interactive information that can help satisfy the increasing demand at negligible cost.

By presenting good-quality information we have the potential to improve our patients' decision making. They can improve their own medical care, make better and more appropriate use of the resources we offer and be made aware of additional treatment options such as self-care. It enhances patient experience and improves use of clinical time. Familiarity breeds reassurance and through the development of the virtual surgery with pictures of the staff, waiting and treatment areas, our patients are no longer visiting an anxiety-provoking, new environment. We can share our recognition of their worries and through this increase our patients' confidence in our practices and can set the doctor–patient relationship off to a good start before the patient arrives at the surgery. It may seem unlikely to us but the waiting room can to many seem a hostile and frightening place and pictures and better information on how our practice systems work can only help.

Still not convinced? Electronic practice information leaflets can reach the 30% plus of people who have Internet access and allow for near instant updates on the changing practice environment – staff changes, holidays, clinics and practice information. Changes to surgery policies, appointment systems and management can be made as they occur, without the cost of stationery design, production and dissemination. We can even produce electronic newsletters to reach out to registered users and have online discussion forums to function as virtual patient-participation groups.

If we create our own links page with links to local and national resources we can encourage our patients towards authoritative medical resources and away from the junk that abounds on the Net. So our patients can be helped to find appropriate information to improve their care and follow up from other healthcare resources. We can use what is one of the most cost-effective communication mediums to promote the practice's view on news and topical issues. We can inform the public on emergency and out-of-hours services and other important local arrangements. The practice website has huge public relations capabilities if we choose to use them to strengthen our professional role and value in the eyes of society. GPs can spin the Web!

If you are of a more commercial bent, why not use it to promote practice services to prospective patients and businesses and to retain existing patients. If you run a travel clinic or perform employment medicals your website can be used to tell patients about these and the charges you make. You don't need much to get on the Web, just:

- a Web address, e.g. http://www.the-gp.co.uk
- Web-authoring software such as FrontPage or Dream-weaver
- Web space
- a Web publishing program.

However, to produce a professional site takes a lot of effort and adding functions such as interactivity and discussion forums can be very time consuming. So the cost is in development time rather than in the tools you need to get on the Web. An effective website needs regular updating so you may well be taking on a significant extra responsibility when you start out as the practice Webmaster. This way of getting on the Web is undoubtedly one for the enthusiast!

The second way is to pay a consultant to develop your website for you. You specify what you require and they design and configure the site to your specification. This can cost upwards of £500 for a site of half a dozen pages, with virtually no upper limit on the amount you could decide to spend. The more pages and functions your site requires the more you will pay. You usually get three or four free content updates a year and you could be charged £50 per page for extra updates. You get a site that will look professional and does what you specify, or you don't pay! This is probably the way to go if you do not think much will change in your practice and you want a hands-off approach, but it may be expensive.

A third way is to use one of a number of companies offering free sites for GPs. Free? We all know, of course, that nothing is free. So these 'free' sites tend to be funded by advertising and, not unreasonably, they usually tie you in to promoting your free site for a number of years so as to attract local business to pay for an advertisement on your site. So read the small print!

Finally, there are template sites produced by organisations such as BT, Sage (http://www.sage.com), who produce generic template sites, and Primary Care Technologies (http://www.healthcentral.co.uk) who produce template sites specifically for primary care. These sites take the HTML programming out of site production and by typing information into online forms it is readily published on the Web without the need for much in the way of technical skill. This method of site production gives the practice a professional site, which can be updated with little trouble and is within the capability of most practices to manage themselves. These start at around £500, are very flexible to use but differ greatly from one another in the facility to individualise the site. It is very easy to get on the Web but a bit harder to create a unique Web presence! Look out for ease of customisation and support with these sites as well as any extra costs for updates – there should not be any!

All these facilities are available now but coming along soon is the ability for patients to book appointments over the Web, order repeat prescriptions and for GPs to conduct electronic consultations by e-mail or live online. Subject of course to stringent security precautions, they are all heralded in the NHS Plan and expected to happen over the next eight years; your practice website is likely to be the doorway through which patients access these services. So maybe the time to seize control of the Web is now before you have to! At least that way you can shape it yourselves.

10
Telemedicine

Telemedicine, it sounds glamorous doesn't it? So glamorous in fact that the Government has put it in the NHS Plan where it must be 'routinely considered in health improvement plans'. Telemedicine is therefore a key part of local implementation strategies (LIS) as well as the national strategy. So what is telemedicine and what part is it really likely to play in the delivery of healthcare in the 21st century? What does your LIS say about it? Telemedicine starts life really as something pretty 'un-glam' and ordinary. The telephone, when used for medicine, is telemedicine at its most commonplace, used every day in every practice. 'Tele' from the Greek meaning 'far off' and 'medicine' derived from the Latin '*mederi*' to heal, so you see it does what it says! Healing from afar. So why all the excitement? Excitement about this, like many things, is often raised because of potential; what we believe may happen or we hope will happen. What we are hoping with telemedicine is that we can deliver existing care programmes more efficiently (cheaply) in a way that is more convenient and acceptable to the consumer (Oops! I must have slipped into thinking I was a politician!). There should also be the potential for patients to receive new types of care because of the remote support potential of telemedicine. As with many dreams, fantasy merges with reality in the high public profile, giving that familiar sensation of spin that one day we may wake from. So, how can the everyday practice draw some practical benefits from telemedicine for its patients?

The phone, a relatively new technology, has revolutionised delivery of healthcare from afar and there is much that new technologies can continue to do in delivery of care from a distance. Take diabetes, for example, and the results of a study by the US military in August 2000 which found that in a study of only 28 patients with insulin dependent diabetes, home consultations by computer helped patients control their blood sugars. The telemedicine group of patients were given computer systems, blood pressure monitors and voice and video communications through the telephone. Virtual visits were conducted by a specialist nurse each week and over three months average blood sugars fell by 16% and weight by 4%. Colonel Alan Mease concluded (in *Military Medicine*, August 2000) that telemedicine technology was a valuable tool in treating diabetes. So too I guess would weekly visits in person by a specialist diabetic nurse but, none the less, telecare works. We can today provide remote access to facilities that might be more expensive to deliver in other ways. It will however take the computer to become as essential a part of life for everyone as the phone is before it benefits more than a very select group in society in this sort of way.

NHS Direct and NHS Direct Online are likely to become the prime sources of delivery of information for patients and their carers in the UK . . . telemedicine as well as telephone triage and it's in a hurry. NHS Direct takes the telephone and uses computer support to enhance the human role. A small number of highly-trained people provide the interface with complex technology on behalf of the masses, a pragmatic application of technology. The interactive website that is its Internet sibling helps step people through a triage system too but requires a moderate level of Internet 'savvy' as well as the cash to get them Internet access. It has the potential to help many people but at the moment those least likely to need it. Of course there *is* an offshore wind and an incoming tide and soon everyone will be in the surf!

Social care and home support and monitoring, much as in the diabetes example, may increase convenience for patients and offer the potential for new diagnostics – the remote ECG linked to a WAP phone perhaps, or maybe a combined device you just press to your precordium that then sends a trace directly to your local cardiologist who can tell you your diagnosis instantly online. That is provided your neck will bend sufficiently for you to get your ear to the phone on your chest! Believe me, this is not as far-fetched as it sounds. Take a look at www.cardiacpen.de. Their device called the Card-iac-pen does almost this. It even has an infrared transmitter which could talk to your notebook PC and send the trace over your mobile. Automated home prompting services, a bit like a computerised personal medical diary where patients are reminded to take their medication or perform their exercises, are imminent. This process takes existing technology and pushes its use a little further.

Videoconferencing is probably what most of us think of when we consider telemedicine. A camera sits on your desk and transmits moving pictures to a specialist sitting in an ivory tower. The specialist tells you to lift the patient's leg or strike their knee with a patella hammer. He then sagely explains the diagnosis that is beyond the ken of a mere GP, and we obligingly issue the prescription and our hugely satisfied patient goes away cured. So why don't we all use videoconferencing rather than refer our patients in the flesh? One reason this dream isn't reality is because of the technology! Currently affordable videoconferencing for GPs means that you get a postage stamp-sized, jerky picture in the corner of your computer screen. This is so small as to be practically useless. The reason for this problem is because of something called bandwidth, or rather the lack of it. Pictures in true colour require huge amounts of data to be sent if the original is to be represented accurately. This means that the pipes that carry this information need to be large bore to squeeze the data down. If you reduce the frequency of information collection you reduce the amount that is sent. That's logical isn't it? This is why you get a jerky image; changes in position of the subject take place that are skipped by the camera but would be discernible to the naked eye. The image appears on screen like some early cine film. The number of slices of data a camera captures are recorded in frames (pictures) per second. Television pictures are displayed at 30 frames per second (fps) and this is probably the standard we need for fluid images. This needs lots of bandwidth. Equally logical is the bigger the image the more data required to transmit the image. So if you only send a small image you can get by with a smaller pipe, hence the postage stamp image we see in the corner of the screen. If, however, you can sit on the data like an overstuffed suitcase you can obviously get more in the package. So data compression techniques, the bum on the suitcase of image manipulation, mean that you can transmit smaller packets that contain the same information over any pipe of a given size.

Even with modern compression, ISDN is undoubtedly the minimum any of us needs for half way acceptable videoconferencing; the pipe size is 64 K, only just bigger than is achievable with a modem (56 K). That is not good enough. Fortunately, standard ISDN contains two pipes of this size, which can effectively be bonded together to provide the equivalent of a single 128 K pipe. So the first thing to do if this technology tempts you is to make sure you can use both of your NHSnet ISDN connection channels (pipes) bonded together. At the moment most of us cannot, so to get this enabled we need to talk to the PCG or health authority. Do it today!

You will need a camera capable of 30 fps, image compression software and probably hardware too. The camera may be inexpensive but, as with most IT, the most important thing for practical use is the appropriate software, which can be expensive, particularly if a specialist medical solution is used. The advantage of the latter is that it should contain integral encryption technology, which makes the communication of this patient-identifying information secure. The other thing you need is compatible software at the other end of the link. This is about communication after all!

More difficult than that is getting someone else at the end of the link when you are at your end, as the videoconference happens live. You need patient and GP (or nurse) at one end and specialist at the other. The consequence is that teleconsultations are expensive in terms of time and human resources consumed. They probably only become viable when there is extensive geographical separation. Hence Norway is a leader in telemedicine and in the UK teleconsulting is most likely to be used in the Highlands and Islands and other remote areas, or where superspecialist services render face-to-face consultations difficult. The presence of high bandwidth and inexpensive high-quality cameras and simple software with the ubiquity of the telephone will change this from being an exceptional technology to a normal part of consultations both between patients and GPs and GPs and specialists. Although this may still seem a long way off, it is definitely on the horizon with the advent of videophones and bandwidth provided by ADSL, and will add a new medium for communication as revolutionary as was the telephone.

In the shorter term, use of videoconferencing in practices has considerable potential for enhancing educational opportunities, allowing real-time clinical conferences and grand rounds to take place in the surgery. IMSI (www.imsi.com) has software that can bring up to 100 attendees to one virtual conference at one time, so the potential of this tool for continuing medical education is tremendous. You put your hand up and the lecturer clicks you onto the screen to make your point or ask a question. The 98 others can all see you and the Prof! Why don't you get your friendly drug company to sponsor a videoconferencing suite in your practice? Get them to put one in your local outpatient department too whilst they are at it!

Quick hits in telemedicine?

Telepsychiatry may seem an anathema to many but how often have you seen a psychiatrist physically examine a patient? Ninety-five per cent of the diagnosis is obtained from the history and observing the patient. This is what teleconsulting allows par excellence and a video-conferencing unit might be used by the CPN and GP as well for case conferences. Once you have one think of what else you might use it for.

A picture speaks a thousand words, does it not, so to add a picture to a dermatology referral letter may in many circumstances allow a diagnosis to be made without the patient physically having to attend the outpatient depart-ment. Saving time for the patient and the specialist, but sadly not for the poor GP. Unless, that is, it shortens waiting lists and reduces the numbers of patients returning to the consulting room to complain about their skin or about the long wait for assessment . . . We live in hope. Static images are also a great follow-up tool for skin problems and for communicating information within the practice. If these are digital images they can be stored on the computer, available to everyone in the practice and attached to an e-mail referral in an instant. The hardware and software to do this is increasingly affordable and is well within the budget of most practices.

Most practices have ECG machines and use them frequently both in acute illness and as a baseline for conditions such as hypertension and for making the diagnosis of arrhythmias. The problem I find is that while I can recognise gross pathology, subtleties often escape me. I am not alone in this. In my practice we send all ECGs to our local cardiologist for reporting after assessing them ourselves. This helps keep us used to interpreting ECGs and enables ongoing education from the positive and negative correlation with the specialist opinion we receive. An electronic recording has considerable benefits, one of which is the fact that you send a copy. The reporting cycle is accelerated and copies can easily be attached to referrals. I would say that if you are investing in a new ECG machine it must be capable of digital output. Speak to your local accident and emergency department and ask them how often access to an old ECG would aid their patient management. If you had a digital copy you could send one instantly and save significant numbers of overnight stays that depend on serial ECGs.

Until now I have really just considered the outward transmission of information from the practice, but tele-radiology opens up a rich seam of information for the practice. Most of us became familiar with looking at X-rays, ultrasounds and even MRI scans when in training. As soon as we enter general practice we are deprived of access to these images. We rely on written reports to explain findings to our patients. Now we could have the images as well as the reports sent to us. A patient comes in with cervical arthritis and we could show them a picture of their own neck on our screen. We might even be able to compare it with the picture of the average cervical spine for someone of that age. Not only do we get the satisfaction of continuing to use our vestigial radiology skills but patients always appreciate *seeing* what is the matter with them. This may not affect the quantity of our work but, as it certainly enriches the quality, it has to be worth considering.

cal practice

With networks in practices and the so-
called of GP clinical systems that support
these new ive an opportunity to increase the
richness and thereiore the value of the clinical record.
Instead of a simple textual Electronic Health Record there
is the facility to attach and integrate pictures, data from
investigations and now sound and even video with the
record. We have the potential not only to store our
description of findings but a visual and auditory record too.

I have mentioned some of the benefits telecardiology can
offer to practices. The following brief list exemplifies some of
the immediate and practical benefits we can get from storing
data digitally:

- recordings are easily stored, retrieved and exchanged
- less physical storage space is required
- data is accessible from all PCs in a network
- individual access rights can be defined
- recordings can easily be compared
- software tools are available for data analysis, e.g. of ECG
  database statistics
- it is well-suited for use in education and training.

All you need to make this work in your practice is an ECG

machine that can export its data to a PC and the appropriate software to manage this. Fortunately all but the most basic modern ECG machines now come with this functionality and you should be able to get something to do the job for around £2000. Modern software can even facilitate one record being graphically overlain on another to vividly illustrate changes, and sophisticated reporting and interpretive functions are integral to most modern software. You also need a GP system that can support the linking of this digital information to the patient record. If you have a Windows-based system then this will almost certainly be the case. If you still have a text-based system then there are often ways of attaching such digital files to the EPR. If not, don't despair; if you just stock your system with the digital information then when you have a clinical computer that can cope with digital attachments the ECG can be associated with the patient's record. Historical ECGs can be of great use in deciding when a change has occurred, and have considerable implications for patient care. ST elevation in a trace that was not present a couple of years ago can mean the difference between admitting someone to coronary care or keeping them at home. Therefore there can be considerable value in thinking ahead and storing the digital information for a time when it may develop greater value.

Some products are available that are effectively software ECGs. The limb and chest leads just plug into a USB socket on your PC, all the calculations are done in the PC's processor and your laser or inkjet printer is used for making a hard copy. This usually means that a 12-lead ECG can be printed out on a single side of A4 or customised to fit neatly into a Lloyd George envelope. To get added telemedicine functions additional software may be required at the receiving end that supports ECG record display and third-party reporting. Software compatibility may be an issue as different standards exist and, unlike JPEG and TIFF standards for images, the viewers for which are free or an integral part of most operating systems (Windows, Linux, UNIX etc), the specialist nature of ECGs means that proprietary systems are common. You need to be sure that before you spend a couple of grand on an ECG it is compatible with that used by your local cardiology department, so that you can take advantage of the communication potential of telecardiology.

Digital photography

This is probably the quickest hit from telemedicine and digital information storage. Costs are low and the benefits are visible. Take the teenage lad with acne. He attends the surgery having tried all the over-the-counter treatments to no avail. Before you had the digital camera you might have recorded moderate/severe acne with comedones and pits on the face and shoulders. Then three months later, after a course of tetracyclines, you might record the patient's opinion that it was no better and your own that there had been slight improvement. The teenager, fed up with his acne, overestimates its severity. We, with our desire to produce improvement through our treatment, overestimate its efficacy. Now you have a camera and you can see the improvement or lack of it because three months of waiting has not clouded the picture as it may cloud memory. Not only that but if the patient comes back to see your partner, not you, they have a true record of progress and effectiveness of treatment and are in a much better position to decide on the next stage of treatment. Some practices have used Polaroid (http://www.polaroid.co.uk) cameras for this purpose for years but films were expensive and only a single copy would be made. Digital cameras produce instant pictures that can be copied, forwarded and shared. You can even e-mail your patient a copy! All at no cost above that of the digital camera.

It is not just GPs who benefit. In many practices nurses

laboriously trace the size of leg ulcers to monitor their tedious course to resolution. This is very time consuming. A picture makes an excellent record. All that is required is the camera and a standard scale or grid to place against the lesion and an accurate record is made in an instant. Subtleties such as colour and texture are recorded too, enhancing the value of this record whilst saving time for your nurses. So that's at least two cameras you will need!

A highly sophisticated refinement of the digital camera is digital fundoscopy. Cameras now exist that can take retinal images through the undilated pupil and produce superb images on screen. Far in advance of anything the mortal GP can see through even a well-dilated pupil. There is now stacks of evidence to show that retinal photography and direct fundoscopy combine to provide the gold standard for managing diabetic eye disease, and not dilating pupils means that the procedure is faster as well as more accurate. If you combine this with increased acceptability to our patients as now they can drive home afterwards, it seems hard to justify not using this superb tool. Err . . . it costs around £20 000 for the hardware and software. Could that be the justification for not using it? Possibly, but one computerised fundoscopy unit for the PCG, or one shared between practices, would make a lot of sense and is a first-rate example of the value of information technology, especially as the result can be squirted down the phone line to our ophthalmologist colleagues for a second opinion whenever we are in doubt.

Spirometers can likewise produce digital output, which can be used to add detailed respiratory function results to the electronic record or the image of the full spirometry chart attached to the record. Sphygmomanometers may also be used to enter information directly into the record but template manual entry is very fast and the only gain from doing it automatically is to avoid transcription errors on data entry.

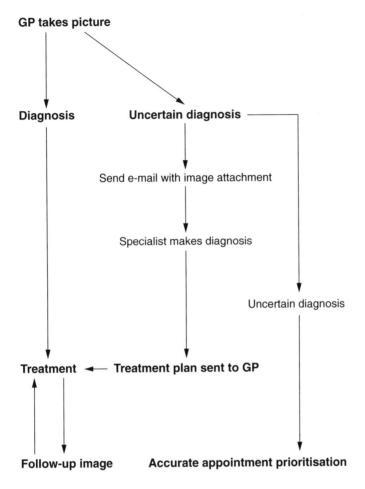

Figure 11.1 Typical sequence in a patient management system using digital images.

NHS Direct Online

NHS Direct Online is a Government-funded website that provides health information in the format of electronic leaflets and interactive systems. The latter take you through questions until you reach your diagnosis, treatment option or both with the security of a phone number for NHS Direct for ear-to-ear consultation by phone if you get worried. Access to NHS Direct Online can be gained through any Internet connection but there are plans for NHS Direct Online kiosks to be installed in public places and larger surgeries might well start pushing their health authority or PCG to install one. Touch-sensitive screens and simple menu displays are very user friendly and need not require much practice involvement to support the access process.

Computerised cognitive behavioural therapy (CBT) is another digital service your practice could offer to patients. It sounds bizarre doesn't it, something as personal as behavioural therapy for depression and anxiety being delivered by computer? Behavioural therapy does work; the problem is that there are just not enough therapists and even if there were it is immensely time consuming for the therapist and therefore immensely expensive. We just could not afford it for all of our patients who might benefit. This is not a unique situation for this or any other healthcare system. But there is now a choice. Hal, our friendly stand-alone PC in 2001, can deliver effective CBT. Beating the Blues (http://www.ultrasis.com) is a program produced at the Institute of Psychiatry by Dr Judy Proudfoot. It delivers a course of eight sessions lasting just less than an hour each. Think what that would cost if delivered by a psychologist. It takes you through problem identification, goal setting, thinking disorders and how to overcome them, looking at attributional style, the way we explain things to ourselves and helps re-set these into a healthier pattern. In other words, it leads the patient through standard best practice in CBT and enables the treatment of large number of patients with minimal demand on clinical time. It does, of course, produce hard copy reports at the end of each session, which can be kept by the patient or retained in the medical record. Such applications of technology add a new dimension to the therapeutic armamentarium and may well attract the more touchy-feely amongst us into using IT where otherwise it would hold little appeal.

Interactive programs for management of chronic conditions such as diabetes create new treatment options for patients and ways of reinforcing good practice and self-care. The list goes on for new ways that technology can assist the traditional role of personal medical care. Not as a replacement for clinicians but as tools and adjuncts to conventional treatment that, as with all treatments, work best when used to treat the right patients. Where they win over those established treatments is in reducing expensive clinical input and allowing delivery of specialist intervention by non-specialists. In the NHS environment of cost-efficient delivery of care the potential use of patient-administered software in the practice environment needs consideration. Those of us who are building a new surgery should probably be thinking about where the patient kiosk can be sited, and planning to set up at least one room for computer–patient interaction. This PC, for use by patients, should be stand alone and disconnected from the NHSnet and practice clinical network to prevent breaches of confidentiality or hacking by a disgruntled patient. Nonetheless, I expect patient appointments for computer consultation to become commonplace in many practices in the not too distant future!

12
VoicE

Technology allows us to manage sounds in new ways; VoicE is just a sophisticated series of sounds, and some that are not so sophisticated. The telephone and the computer are getting closer as the analogue transmission of sound information changes to digital. They can now even share the same wiring as our computers. What does that give us? Why an acronym of course, CTI, computer telephone integration, and CTI should not be ignored in the development of the paperless practice. Another area where voice management and evolving technology has the potential to make our lives easier is in the dictation of letters and documents. The latter forms the main part of this chapter but I will first touch upon CTI.

CTI

This is not discussed in much detail but it will give a flavour of what can be done and what the next step is in bringing change about. We tend to buy a phone system and use it until it breaks or stops working due to old age. Yet we expect to replace our computer hardware every three to five years. Why are phones treated differently? Computerised phone systems can give us voicemail with individual mail boxes . . . multiple if we like with one for practice messages, one for professional messages and perhaps even a third for our patients. Messages can be time- and date-stamped and even forwarded to other mailboxes if we are absent from the practice for a more protracted time. All calls can be recorded to improve our security in negligence claims, but remember the need to respect patient confidentiality and to inform all callers that their calls will be recorded. Receptionists can automatically be presented with the medical records of only those patients with that particular number in their records, picking from a list of only half a dozen or so when answering a call. This saves time for patient and practice alike.

Direct dial extensions are no longer the territory of big businesses – we can all have them. Practice managers can receive almost all their calls directly, smoothing workflow in the practice. How about a single extension number for the practice's patient advice line that can be routed to the doctor or nurse responsible for the advice at the time? Or how about medical advice to promote the uptake of flu vaccine by your vulnerable patients and over 65s when callers are put on hold? It's more appropriate than muzak and has the potential to do a lot of good . . . maybe everyone needs to be left on hold for a couple of minutes. The message can be changed in seconds to respond to the latest tabloid anxiety and, if given with the authoritative and friendly voice of their own GP, may cause some patients to proceed no further.

The message is clear: we should review our phone systems regularly every few years. We should try to ensure that the systems we buy are upgradeable, as often all that needs to be changed is the software heart. Telephone systems are highly specialist and we would probably all be well advised to seek expert professional advice. This is where the NHS can help. The NHSIA have a telecoms department with regional experts who can review practice phone systems, advise on how they can be upgraded and even advise on the different systems on the market. Use them, that's what they're there for!

Paperless dictation

There are three areas here that offer some hope of escape from the mountains of paperwork engulfing us. Voice recognition is the sexiest subject; it is possibly still suffering from premature ejaculation, but its time will come (did I get that the right way around?). Network dictation systems and their big brother Internet transcription services take what we do already with tape and integrate it with developing infrastructures in practices and the Internet. It is probably easiest to consider these individually but one part of the technology merges with the other and the solution to our problems is inclusive rather than exclusive.

Network dictation systems

There are some quick gains here for practices from the installation of the practice computer network (LAN, local area network) that accompanies their NHSnet connection. A networked computer system allows the individual PC to see and have access to any or all of the files on any or all of the other PCs on the same network – if they are given the right permissions; I'll show you mine if you show me yours. It also allows you to use other people's bits and pieces, their hard drive or printer for instance. So I could type a letter on the PC in my consulting room that is actually stored on my secretary's PC hard drive. In voice terms this is like having the microphone to your secretary's Dictaphone in your surgery and a virtually endless tape. Everyone on the network has the same facility.

I find it a constant irritation to run out of tapes for my pocket dictation machine. My secretary finds it a constant irritation to get a tape full of dictation that has been produced by me over a week or ten days when she could have typed much of it earlier. My patients would be irritated to know that there has been a delay on their routine referral whilst I fill up the tape. Now I know most of you are more efficient than me in your dictation management but some of you at least must share some of the same problems. Network dictation means you never run out of tape, you can smooth your secretary's workflow and speed the turnaround of referrals and letters. So how do you do it? The big name here is probably familiar to you as it has now entered common parlance – Dictaphone. Another name that is less well known, but more important as it has recently taken over Dictaphone, is Lernout & Hauspie, a Belgian technology company whose speciality is voice recognition.

Network transcription

This is the Internet rearing its head again, I'm afraid. If you can communicate from your desk across the Internet to someone sitting in an office on the other side of the world as quickly as someone in the office next door, and they can take dictation for half the cost and e-mail you back the letter or forward it directly to its intended recipient, why don't you use them? This is the basis of network transcription services. Some of the big guys like Dictaphone, as was, have produced software that allows for the secure wrapping or encryption of digitised voice files, which are then decrypted at a central office or by homeworkers who then manually convert them to text. They then send them back to you. A unique identifier on your system allows the data to be anonymised when sent and re-identified when received back in the practice. As this is currently proposed most of us, I believe, should have concerns about the confidentiality and security of such an arrangement. If, however, this was within our clinical domain or at least within our sphere of influence, such as the PCG who might use a bank of secretaries to manage practice workload more efficiently, it might just be acceptable. So perhaps this is the shape of things to come. Personally, I hope not as my secretary does so much more than transcribe but economic factors may drive us into it.

Voice recognition

Voice recognition usually means that we know the origin of the voice we hear. In IT circles it means something different. It is the translation of voice into a textual representation of the original. Where it does have something in common with the traditional meaning of voice recognition is that to translate effectively, it has to learn the characteristics of the voice to correctly interpret it into meaningful language displayed as text. Voice recognition technology has been considered by many to be the Holy Grail of data entry into computers. Talk to them and they can interpret what you say as it was meant, no need to learn how to control a mouse or use a keyboard – just use the voice and language you learnt as a child.

Such technology is with us now and is being built into the next Office suite and operating system from Microsoft. It can already be used as independent but integrated packages with Microsoft Office, Corel or Lotus products and to control our browsers for surfing the Internet. How can this speech technology be used in the 21st century paperless practice? Well, simply, why write it twice? Adding a second human into the chain of message production that we call letter writing not only wastes time but also adds the potential for increased error, although of course a good secretary picks up your mistakes and brings them to your notice. However, a good wordprocessor can do the same quite easily for both grammar and spelling and if it does not know a word, once you have told it the computer remembers it forever. Or at least until it crashes! That's the other part of speech recognition then . . . a good wordprocessor and vocabulary (dictionary). All speech recognition software comes with both but to cope with our needs it is probably easiest for the editing to be done from within your usual office product.

How does it all work? Well, you speak into a microphone attached to your computer's soundcard. Both of these bits of kit are important, the mike will usually come with your voice recognition software but it is worth investing a few extra pounds in getting the best quality that is compatible. The quality of input affects the recognition and the better the recognition the less time and effort dictating letters takes. The soundcard likewise affects the accuracy of information going into the voice software. *Always* get a soundcard that is on the approved list of the software you are buying. Getting a full list may mean a call to the software support line or a visit to their website but if you are having problems it's time well spent. Your existing hardware may be fine but if you get lots of gobbledegook check the compatibility of these input devices. The soundcard takes the analogue signal from the mike and converts it into a digital format that the software running on your computer can then work its magic on. The price of the magic is, however, high. It makes lots of demands on your system's memory and processor. To convert sounds into text in real time, as you speak, requires enormous numbercrunching power. It is really strange and distracting to see words appear on the screen several minutes after you have spoken them, which is what happens with a slow PC. If this happens to you it's probably easier to dictate without being able to see the screen!

What's your hourly rate? It only takes the equivalent of a wasted hour to buy an extra 32 Mb RAM or a significantly faster processor. Currently, most (voice recognition) software specifies at least a 300 MHz Pentium equivalent processor and 64 Mb of memory. I would advise at least a 500 MHz processor and 128 Mb RAM but as this is now the basic specification starter system, what most of us have on our desks should do the job admirably.

So with a noise-cancelling mike, compatible soundcard and state of the art hardware, you are almost ready to go – but what software do you choose? With this being the Holy Grail you would expect some big names to be involved and you would be right: Microsoft are there partnering Lernout & Hauspie (more of them in a minute), and IBM and Philips are also in the frame. Philips has been involved in this arena for years producing specialist voice products for our radiologist colleagues but they do not at present have a specialist product for GPs. They do have a consumer product called Freespeech. IBM also has a consumer product, Simply Speaking. These are highly competent in spite of their low price. Lernout & Hauspie (L&H) have their Voice Xpress range of products. They also have that of their recent and chief competitor Dragon Systems, called Naturally Speaking. Dictaphone is now also in their stable. That takeover has meant that one company, L&H, are in a very commanding position for your money. How do you choose between them? It's a puzzle and with each system leapfrogging the other in terms of accuracy if I was to recommend one it would have changed by tomorrow. I would, however, use that as your yardstick. Accuracy: it has to come first. It takes time editing and the thing we all want more of is time, so don't waste it. If you are buying for the first time get whatever is most accurate. The software producer's websites will have links to review articles. Find an independent competitive comparison and go for the one that is most accurate: end of story.

All voice recognition software needs a period of training for it to learn your voice and most will improve as you use them and correct errors. If you do not correct your errors the software does not learn from its mistakes and will make them again and again and again *ad infinitum*. Natural speech recognition is now the norm and the staccato created by having to pause between words should no longer be necessary. Once the system has learnt your vocal idio-syncrasies by reading such stimulating passages as 'Mary had a little lamb' or the like, often for quite some time, you have your own individual profile that can be copied to a floppy and used on any machine on which the software is installed. You do of course need multiple licenses for multiple users. Each user has to train the software themselves for the system to build each individual voice profile.

So you can now dictate on any computer that has your profile – but you are not always at a computer. Do not despair, there are now mobile devices just like your usual pocket tape recorder, some may even be your usual pocket recorder. These plug into your PC and automatically upload your dictation, converting your dulcet tones into text before your eyes. Of course, you then have to go through the process of correction and proof reading, but it is pretty impressive. The beauty of this is that you could have multiple mobile digital transcribers and the voice recogni-tion software installed just once on your secretary's PC. Just plug in your handset to her (or his) machine and there it is, your dictation on their machine to edit and proof read. The best of both worlds – your secretary has to correct your errors but the voice recognition software should be able to achieve 95% accuracy and save her lots of time typing. You can send her the file over the practice network or even over the Internet if you have the right software on your local machine.

L&H products have the advantage of a medical vocabu-lary add on. It's not cheap but this helps, as the software does not hiccup every time it hits a new word. Individual specialist medical vocabularies or dictionaries can often be added to any of these products from stand-alone packages at a lower cost. All of these systems will build their own medical vocabularies in time and with use, but the hidden cost of correction needs to be added into the equation when deciding which to buy. It is often possible to get trial software for these programmes from the manufacturer, their websites or even from cover disks on PC magazines, and this is an excellent way of seeing whether you want to buy one product or another. Have a look around to see what is available or would meet your needs best, then buy it!

One last word – there are those who swear by voice recognition and those who swear at it but whichever you are keep your early attempts, they can be hilarious!

13
Security and confidentiality in the digital age

Trust none: For oaths are straws, men's faiths are wafer cakes,
And hold-fast is the only dog, my duck.   (Henry V)

Be afraid, very afraid. The consequences of a breach in security for a practice are immense. The harm that could be caused to patients is similarly immense both from the exposure of individual patient information and from the corruption and destruction of the whole practice record. The surgery might burn down and the notes destroyed by fire or the fireman's flood. 'OK', I can almost hear you say, 'a set of notes might be mislaid whilst visiting and they might turn up on the newsdesk of a local paper. So what is so different now?' Well, by storing our databases of patient information in electronic form we create additional vulnerability, whilst the risk of fire and flood remain.

Physical dangers like lightning and power surges can corrupt and wipe all the patient records, and hard disk failure can do the same. Software can have bugs, and viruses may inadvertently infect our clinical system and lead to its untimely demise. By connecting to the Internet we open a window to the world that was not there before. Electronic eyes can peer at our patients' secrets and we might never know. Electronic fingers could pick through our records and then shuffle them to the point that they are un-useable and slip away untraceably down the wire. A disaffected member of the practice could wipe the hard drive. The old server might be bought at auction with the entire practice database still on the system. The paper equivalent of this for my practice would be for me to leave 8500 Lloyd George envelopes on my car roof and drive off. Even I am unlikely to do that but I can imagine leaving the laptop with just the same information on it beside the car and driving off, with disastrous consequences.

While having computerised medical records makes patients' records more secure from some risks, at the same time they are rendered more vulnerable to others. Sometimes the very effect of computerisation is to achieve these two opposites. For instance, offsite back-up, taking the weekly back-up tape home, substantially reduces the risk of losing the bulk of patient records if there is a serious fire at the surgery, but this duplication doubles the risk of records accidentally getting into the public domain. On other occasions there are distinct gains from computerisation in terms of the security of clinical records. A letter sent by post may be delivered to the wrong address or be opened by the wrong person, whereas an encrypted e-mail can only be unlocked and read by its intended recipient and even show whether it has been tampered with en-route. It's a much harder prospect to identify an envelope that has been steamed open and resealed, which is the paper equivalent. So how do we navigate the shark-filled waters of data security and confidentiality?

People issues

Dame Fiona Caldicott was charged with producing guidance on security and confidentiality of medical records and has produced detailed principles on how this should be achieved. The key principles on patient information it enshrines should be in everyone's mind.

Box 13.1 The Caldicott principles

Principle 1: justify the purpose(s)
Every proposed use or transfer of patient-identifiable information within or from an organisation should be clearly defined and scrutinised, with continuing uses regularly reviewed by an appropriate guardian.

Principle 2: don't use patient-identifiable information unless it is absolutely necessary
Patient-identifiable information items should not be used unless there is no alternative.

Principle 3: use the minimum necessary patient-identifiable information
Where use of patient-identifiable information is considered to be essential, each individual item of information should be justified with the aim of reducing identifiability.

Principle 4: access to patient-identifiable information should be on a strict 'need to know' basis
Only those individuals who need access to patient-identifiable information should have access to it, and they should only have access to the information items that they need to see.

Principle 5: everyone should be aware of their responsibilities
Action should be taken to ensure that those handling patient-identifiable information – both clinical and non-clinical staff – are aware of their responsibilities and obligations to respect patient confidentiality.

Principle 6: understand and comply with the law
Every use of patient-identifiable information must be lawful. Someone in each organisation should be responsible for ensuring that the organisation complies with legal requirements.

The key points can be more easily remembered by using FIONA C:

- Formal justification of purpose
- Information transferred only when absolutely necessary
- Only the minimum required
- Need to know access controls
- All to understand their responsibilities
- Comply with and understand the law.

(John Griffin, Thames Gateway)

Another acronym that identifies the key areas is CIA, Confidentiality, Integrity, Authenticity: you knew it stood for that, didn't you?

- Confidentiality is our duty to keep information within the circle of trust acceptable to the patient.
- Integrity is our duty to keep the information safe from loss or unauthorised change.
- Authenticity is to ensure that the information is ascribed to and created by the person(s) who purport to have created it. Remember the CIA as we go along.

All health organisations have to appoint a Caldicott guardian; in a practice this is likely to be the practice manager, a GP or senior nurse. It is this person's responsibility to look after information security and confidentiality, both paper and electronic. As one of their first tasks they should draw up an information security policy for the practice and as the health authority and PCG must have a Caldicott guardian too, there should be support and advice available. All practice staff will need training to ensure they know their own responsibilities with regard to patient confidentiality and medical records. Suggest that your PCG runs training days, maybe. Where the practice gives access to attached staff employed by another organisation, thought must be given as to how their training and awareness of data security in the practice is addressed and, of course, who foots the bill for it!

Who actually enters the information on the computer system? In many practices there will be partners who do not and will not acquire the necessary skills to make the record themselves, and others where it is the established practice to dictate or pass notes of visits or other consultations to a clerk to enter into the patient record. Here is an authenticity issue. The audit trail will identify the individual entering data but the record must identify the person responsible for eliciting that information and responsible for that clinical intervention. The accuracy and completeness of the record are part of its integrity and clinicians may be held liable for information entered for them. All entries should:

1 normally be made by the person responsible for the information recorded

2 record who entered the information

3 record the time, date and place of data entry

4 be entered during the consultation or as soon as possible afterwards

5 be audited regularly for accuracy and completeness where entries are made by a third party.

Physical issues: fire, flood, theft, power failure, lightning strike

What is 'physical' when you are talking of computer records? Some things are obvious, like keeping the computer in a safe place, others are less so, like protection from fire and flood. The former are all too frequently followed by the latter! Others are still more obtuse, like the risk of computer viruses and the destruction of hard disks. Whatever the threat the least important issue is damage to the kit and the most important is the safety of patient information. So let us start with back-up.

Back-ups should be done regularly. For most practices the minimum is on a daily basis but as our dependence on computer systems increases, so we should consider more frequent back-ups. These should be cycled through every week with a weekly and monthly back-up in case of virus attack or data corruption, so that it is possible to go back to a known good record. One thing that has caught practices out is when back-ups appear to have taken place but there has been no transfer of data or the data will not restore from the tape. The risk of this is reduced by the use of good-quality software but it is probably wise to send data tapes to your GP system supplier, by secure courier of course, every couple of months to check (a) that all the data is there and (b) that it can be restored. Back-up media should be stored securely in a fireproof safe away from the main premises. Establishing these processes will normally be the responsibility of your very own practice Caldicott guardian.

The use of redundancy in GP system disk storage may help ensure we always have access to our electronic records. Hot, swappable disks that allow the computer to continue running in spite of the failure of one of its disks, and the disk to be replaced without system downtime, are becoming necessities for the larger paperless practices. However, it is wise to check that the nirvana of no downtime, is actually the case when a disk fails. My experience is that even with hot, swappable RAID (random array of inexpensive disks) systems there is inevitably downtime as the disks write to both disks at the same time. If there is only one to write to they don't like it and stop functioning. Horribly techie, isn't it? But as 80% of system failures are down to hard disk problems, attention to this area is well worth the effort.

Box 13.2 Theft minimisation

General

- Have a secure building – locks, alarms, etc.
- Locate server and PCs out of public view.
- Security mark all IT equipment.
- Record serial numbers of all PCs.
- Keep the main server in a locked room or cabinet.
- Fix freestanding computers to the floor or piece of solid furniture; many now come with a loop for a chain specifically for this purpose.

Laptops

- Never leave in open view in an unattended vehicle.
- Remove all patient-identifiable information regularly.
- Back-up clinical information to the GP system as soon as is practicable after the consultation.
- Password protect the laptop log on.
- Encrypt all information on the hard disk.
- Install and regularly update virus checking software.

MI5 once left a laptop containing confidential information in a taxi after a night on the tiles. So, if they can be careless with information, anyone can. Please don't forget your PDAs (personal digital assistants), those natty little hand-held devices from Psion, Palm and the like. These should be treated like laptops and password protection of log on should be a *sine qua non*.

God Himself is not secure, having given man dominion over His
work.   (Helen Keller)

Lightning is a real risk to your electronic patient information
as are other causes of electrical spikes. Your server should be
protected by a UPS (uninterruptible power source), which
can keep the practice system running for at least long
enough to save current information in the event of power
failure. It will also protect the server from surge damage
such as a lightning strike to overhead power lines. To try to
prevent damage to your PCs and information on your hard
drive, get a surge protection device fitted to your power
supply; they only cost a few pounds and are simply installed
by plugging them into the electrical outlet. Socket to me!
(And you probably.)

No matter how safe we make the computer, even if we
lock it in a temperature-controlled room a Jumbo's wing-
span from its mirrored twin system, a virus can kill them
both and destroy data, even in back-ups infected before the
malignant phase. So virus protection is essential. It is more
than calling on the latest software as someone somewhere
always gets hit by the newest bug before it is incorporated
into the protection software. How do we minimise the risk
of that someone being us? We need a virus protection
policy and procedures (see Box 13.3). Viruses spread from
fomites like floppy disks, computers that have been
repaired or even the software installed by your friendly
GP systems engineer. I caught Melissa, my first virus
(strictly she's a worm), from the NHS Information Authority, downloaded from a document on NHSnet – proving
Helen Keller right! This virus hit millions of computers, so
much as I'd like to I can't harbour a grudge.

Getting the physical layout of the building and position of
terminals and computers right does a lot to prevent
inadvertent disclosure of information. Are screens posi-
tioned so that members of the public can easily see them?

Box 13.3 Recommended points for inclusion in a virus protection policy

- All software used on the practice system should be authorised by the Caldicott guardian.
- Don't allow programs to be downloaded from the Internet except by specific authorised users and only onto computers with the latest virus software.
- Set the Microsoft viewer programs as default programs to open e-mail attachments, as unlike the full thing they cannot run macro viruses.
- Run a virus check on all PCs that have been out of the practice domain before re-connecting them to the network.
- Install up-to-date virus-checking software on all laptops that may be connected to the practice system.
- Ask technicians when they last checked their systems for viruses before running any programs on the practice system.
- Update your virus program regularly; many now automate updates from the Internet.

The reception desk is probably the place where this is most likely to occur. Consider physically fixing the position of the screen so that it cannot inadvertently be turned to give patients making an appointment a better view. Thin (TFT) screens may offer less-clear side views of their content, as well as saving space and generating less heat – both added advantages. In the consulting room it is very easy to be called out to an emergency or other pressing problem. Leaving the terminal logged on may allow disclosure of every part of the clinical system. Ensure that there is an easy way to log off and back on again. Making access difficult is probably the best way to prevent inadvertent disclosure.

The issue of access control is one that most of us are aware of through the use of passwords to access the clinical system.

We know these should be kept confidential and changed regularly. Just how regularly however is difficult as the greater the frequency of change the more likely the user is to forget it, or fear forgetting it, and breach security by writing it down or using something obvious. Passwords should generally consist of at least six characters and contain both letters and numbers. It's amazing how many people go blank when asked to provide one. Help them by suggesting they think of a phrase or quotation that is easy to remember, or how about a song or film title with a number in the middle? Screensavers are another simple way of hiding what's on the screen of a PC and can be password protected from Windows 95 onwards. These can be timed to come on if there is no keyboard activity for a specified time . . . at the reception desk, two minutes may be about right. Automating protection works to computers' strengths of err . . . doing things automatically, and can support us frail users.

Levels of access control should vary with different members of the team. Such controls restrict inveterate tamperers like me from doing harm and can improve confidentiality. Remember, if you have Tony Blair and Cherie on your list there are people who would pay a lot of money to access their records, and such records probably require a special security setting. In the secure practice, it is going to be much easier to bribe someone who has legitimate access to turn a blind eye so the intruder can finger through the electronic record, rather than hack your system. They can view the record, make no changes and leave without any record in the audit trail apart from a log on to the system. Access control to sensitive information is much more likely to become an issue in the average practice where members of the team are also patients. In Hampshire, a nurse discovered the results of her laboratory investigations taken by her GP on the Bedfordshire Trust system, there for all her colleagues to see. How will the practice cope with this where staff members, partners too perhaps, are patients?

Special high-level access is undoubtedly required. And what about when staff leave the practice . . . naturally you cancel their access and change any group password they knew, don't you? Or do you?

Wherever there is a printer in a practice there will be waste that is likely to contain confidential material, even if it's just a mangled prescription that got chewed up when printing. Make sure that beside each printer there is a 'confidential' bin whose waste is disposed of securely. One of the most important acquisitions for the paperless practice will be an industrial grade shredder that can cope with the mass of paper that will continue to come into the practice and need destroying. The likelihood of someone trying to get hold of confidential information directly relates to its market value. So, the more sensational the information and the more well-known its subject, the more likely someone is to go through your bins to find the gore on the celeb you saw in your morning surgery, and the worse it will be for you if it happens. If in doubt, shred it!

Inadvertent disclosure can easily take place when a computer disk is replaced or an old PC sold. Destroy the data. I have heard of GPs cooking disks in ovens, freezing them (well it works for resetting my car radio but it won't destroy the data on your disk though) and hitting them with sledgehammers. The last may work but is not as certain as running software that wipes the disk clean and makes information irretrievable. Do not think that simply deleting files by emptying the re-cycle bin is good enough. Files remain on the hard drive and there are probably thousands of 13-year-olds who have the software to retrieve them. Software to remove these files completely is available from Norton (http://www.norton.com) and McAfee; the latter's FileWipe product is generally inexpensive. The message has to be to use the right tool for the job and wipe the disk before disposing of all old PCs.

Security, the Internet and NHSnet

The vast majority of practices in the country have a link from their clinical systems to Racal Healthlink for transmitting claims information. So now we are connecting to NHSnet, why the big fuss about security? That is a question I have been asked several times. The difference is huge. Of course the Racal connection opened a small window onto the practice system through which a hacker could crawl, but that window was into a single room in another building whose doors were bolted and protected by security guards, and only a couple of known and trusted visitors would be allowed in. If there were to be a security breach with Racal, surely it would be an inside job. The NHSnet, by contrast, is not a room but a metropolis. It is an organisation of more than a million people; predominantly good, but a few bad and ugly. NHSnet opened the window to that walled metropolis and put security guards (firewalls) at its few gateways. This, we were told, would keep the hostile banditos of the Internet out and our practice systems would be safe. The problem was that there are a million people inside the walls and, remember, some are ugly. Fortunately, along came Lee van Cleef in the form of the BMA who insisted that practices should employ their own security guards to stand at their windows to keep the baddies out and let the goodies in. This security guard is known as a firewall. This is a bit of software or both software and hardware that filters information from permitted sources only. Only those bits of data that pass the security requirements set in the firewall are then allowed through to the practice network. Firewalls generally require specialist setting up or come with a rigid set-up for an out-of-the-box solution to keep the hackers out.

Our Internet-enabled PCs we have at home require open communication systems for 'talking' over the Internet and without this facility we would be unable to upload and download data over the Internet or send Internet e-mail. However, these open systems leave all communication exposed and renders our system open to hackers who use scanning devices to question hundreds of ISP addresses at random until they find an open socket. When they find one, look out! There is the potential to use this in a malicious way to steal data, corrupt it or use your system to send spam or viruses using your identity.

So why don't we all need firewalls? Increasingly, the answer is actually you probably will. Certainly with the implementation of ADSL technology, which allows for communication ten times faster than the fastest modem over your current BT line, you must. At the moment however most ISPs (BT Internet, AOL, Virgin and Co.) give you a temporary address when you are online. When you hang up they can then re-assign the same address to someone else. This means that Horrible Hacker only has the time that you are online to find you and scan your open sockets and get in. As soon as you log off he has to start that random scanning process again. So, the longer you are online, the more vulnerable you are to hackers and the greater the need for a personal firewall. With ADSL your connection is always on so old HH can spend as long as he likes probing your ports until he finds a way in, unless, that is, you have a firewall. Not only does the firewall prevent the attack but it can alert you to HH trying to sneak in. You can then take action to become more secure and reduce the risk of this and future attacks. Some firewalls even have a defensive sting and can tie the marauding software in knots!

This issue of firewall protection from the Internet is one reason why you have to complete an acceptable user policy (AUP) when you sign-up for connection to NHSnet. If you open your own connection to the Internet by logging on from your PC when you are also connected to the practice system, you have opened a window to a room that also has a window open to NHSnet. In through your window crawls Horrible, into your PC and out through the other window you left open. He then has free range to wander over NHSnet. It's pretty obvious therefore why we need to commit to the NHS security policy. It is equally obvious that within an NHS of a million people someone will inadvertently breach the policy. So we do need good old Lee van Cleef's advice to have a second line of security and have a firewall at practice level.

Cleef (or should that be clef) also holds the key to safe communication of patient-identifiable information over NHSnet. The BMA has said that all such information must be encrypted. That means it is rendered into a form that can only be made sense of by its intended recipient. It does this by creating a large random number, the key, which is then fed to an alligator. I bet that woke you up! No, the large random number, together with your referral letter, is actually fed to an algorithm. Which, the dictionary tells me, is a process or rule for making a calculation. It then jumbles them together and what went in as meat and bread comes out as sausages, and we are all certain that we never know what's in a sausage! The clever bit is that if someone else has the same sausage machine (algorithm and key) and they shove the sausage back in at the bottom, they get your original meat and bread out of the top! That's known as symmetric encryption and for messaging it requires both sending and receiving parties to know the secret key and use the same algorithm, aka sausage machine.

The problem is that most often we want to send secure messages to someone without exchanging sausage machines. I want to send my referral letter to a urologist without meeting them and to verify who they are without prior trust. This makes symmetric encryption impossible. The process requires the use of two keys. I take my referral letter and get the urologist's public key from a computer called a key server . . . anyone can get it. I place these two ingredients in the algorithm together with my own private key, which only I know and, hey presto, sausages! To reconstitute the meat and bread of the message however, the urologist's private key and my public key are required. When the message arrives, the urologist's private key, which only she knows, performs the first part of the decryption on the bit that was encrypted with her public key. At the same time her software automatically collects my public key from the key server and performs the second part of the decryption process on my private key, thus revealing it was genuinely me who sent the referral. Clever, huh? This is known as asymmetric encryption, using a public key system known as RSA (named after Rivest, Shamir and Adleman). This is the sort of system that the NHS will use to encrypt patient-identifiable messages. It should be an almost transparent process for the practice when implemented. It will, however, require the practice to know a little about encryption and management of its keys. It is also another step in messaging that can go wrong and the practice will need to know who to go to if messages cannot be decrypted . . . this will usually be the GP system supplier.

Patient confidentiality RIP

Encryption works and the longer the key the more secure it becomes, so secure in fact that it even frightens governments. The USA banned the export of strong encryption until it realised in January 2000 that it was not only the USA who could produce it. The UK government has learnt from this and has made refusal to disclose your private key a criminal offence punishable with up to two years imprisonment. Worse still is that pleas of having forgotten the key or not knowing it are equally punishable. Even worse still is that it is also an offence to reveal that you have been required to disclose your key. Clinical information is not exempt from this. The reason cited for this power is so that criminals will not use encryption for secure communication. Presumably a drug trafficker facing a potential ten-year prison sentence when challenged to decrypt an e-mail will say 'Oh No! Not two years inside. Here's the evidence Officer' and hand over the key.

The risks from these powers are immense. A benign state can become malign. Medical records can be used to aid genocide, e.g. the Nazis used medical records to identify Jews during the Holocaust. What would have happened in Yugoslavia if Slobodan Milosovicz had had access to medical records on the potential scale of those available within the NHS? That we have government assurance that this will never happen is about as useful as saying that there is no risk to humans from eating BSE-infected beef. It was a previous government who said that and it was a previous government that lied. So with the passage of the Regulation of Investigatory Powers (RIP) Bill, medical confidentiality may have been sent to its grave.

Our security is not a matter of weapons alone. The arm that wields them must be strong; the eye that guides them must be clear and the will that directs them indomitable.

(Franklin D Roosevelt)

Glossary

Algorithm	A detailed set of rules to solve a problem.
Application	A computer program designed to perform a certain task, e.g. wordprocessor.
Archiving	The storage of older, rarely required data in a cheaper and/or more compact form; for an automated system, this usually means putting 'online' data 'offline'.
Back-up	A copy of the data stored in a computer system for use in case of damage to the stored data; also a verb for the act of creating the back-up.
Bandwidth	The amount of data that can be transmitted across a communication channel over a certain period of time.
Browser	A program used to look at World Wide Web documents; Mosaic was the first popular browser, and Netscape Navigator and Microsoft Explorer are currently competing for market leader.
Caldicott	Dame Fiona, who led a review into the use of patient-identifiable information and made recommendations on appropriate safeguards to govern access and storage of that information.
Certification	The issuing of certificates for verifying that people really are who they say they are; a certificate is a public key signed with the private key of a trusted third party.
Client-server	A relationship between two computers in a network (client and server) which defines the roles of each computer.

Clinical governance	A framework through which NHS organisations are accountable for continuously improving the quality and effectiveness of their services.
Digital signature	Cryptographical mechanisms that are used to authenticate the source of transmitted data and to ensure that the person for whom the transmitted data was intended is the only one who can read it. This involves the use of a public and private key.
Disaster recovery	The act of restoring normal computer function after a system failure or data loss.
Domain name	A domain name defines a unique address on the Internet for an organisation, company or individual (e.g. www.healthcentral.co.uk).
Download	Refers to the process of transferring a software package or a computer folder or file from a server to one's own computer.
Electronic data interchange (EDI)	Exchange of data electronically between healthcare applications; standards in the transfer of data are essential for successful EDI, e.g. EDIFACT.
Electronic health record (EHR)	This is the term used to describe the concept of a longitudinal record of a patient's health from the cradle to the grave. It contains and combines subsets of information associated with episodes of care held in EPRs.
Electronic mail (e-mail)	A message sent from one computer user over a network to another computer user; used as a noun and verb in both singular and plural forms.
Electronic patient record (EPR)	A record that contains a patient's personal details, their diagnosis and details about their treatment and assessments undertaken by a clinician; typically it pertains to that from a single clinical institution.
Encryption	Any procedure used in cryptography to

	convert plain text into cipher text in order to prevent any but the intended recipient from reading that data.
File format	Files are created in different formats for reading by different pieces of software, e.g. *.doc, *.txt, *.pdf, *.jpg.
Firewall	Hardware, software or a combination of both that protects a network from unauthorised access while allowing authorised access.
Graphical user interface (GUI)	The use of pictures rather than just words to represent the input and output of a program.
Hard copy	Readable output from a computer generated in a storable form such as printed on paper.
Health informatics	The discipline that deals with the collection, storage, retrieval, communication and optimal use of health-related data, information and knowledge.
Homepage	The entry point of a website.
Hypertext mark-up language (HTML)	The language used to 'mark up' text documents so that they can be formatted appropriately and linked to other documents for use on the World Wide Web.
Interactive services digital network (ISDN)	A special type of phone line that supports faster transmission of data than standard phone lines, e.g. 64 kilobytes/second.
Internet service provider (ISP)	An organisation or company that offers connections to the Internet and support for Internet services such as the World Wide Web.
Intranet	A computer network, based on Internet technologies, that covers an organisation or group of individuals.
Local area network (LAN)	A network within an organisational domain such as a general practice.

Link	A connection between two documents on the Web, usually specified by an anchor in an HTML document.
MIQUEST	A software package designed to extract anonymised health data from GP systems.
Modem	A device that converts digital data that is in a form compatible with computer manipulation to a form that is compatible with telephone equipment for transmission to remote computer equipment, and *vice versa*.
Multimedia	A presentation or document that uses multiple media such as video, still images, sound and text.
National Health Service Information Authority (NHSIA)	A recently formed special health authority charged with managing information and information systems in the NHS; it replaced the IMG.
National service framework (NSF)	Evidence-based standards setting out what patients can expect to receive from the NHS in major disease or care areas.
NHSnet	A communications network designed to support electronic communications for the NHS. An Intranet for the NHS.
NHS Strategic Tracing Service (NSTS)	A service provided for the NHS but not GPs to obtain NHS numbers for individual patients.
NHS trust	A statutory body providing NHS hospital or community care.
Realtime	The processing of transactions as they are being created, e.g. computer monitoring of intensive care patients, computer control of industrial processes.
Requirements for accreditation (RFA)	A set of standards against which GP systems are assessed. It is used to decide which systems may be eligible for reimbursement under GMS.

Search engine	A computer program to search for information held by computers on the World Wide Web, e.g. Alta-Vista, Excite.
Security	The means by which 'privacy' and 'confidentiality' are assured in computer systems; security includes techniques for protecting the data from accidental disclosure, deliberate inspection and physical harm.
SMTP	Simple mail transfer protocol – a communications protocol designed to transfer mail reliably and efficiently across the Internet.
SNOMED (CT)	Systematised nomenclature of human and veterinary medicine – initially developed for the classification of pathology specimens. It is a comprehensive nomenclature for indexing the entire medical record combined with Read Codes as SNOMED CT (clinical terms).
Telemedicine	The delivery of healthcare services at a distance using telecommunication devices, e.g. facsimile, video and audio conferencing.
Terminal	The device for data entry and/or data output, usually without any processing capacity, hard drive etc. (equates to dumb terminal).
Uniform resource locator (URL)	Specification for identifying any file on the Internet. The URL is made up of the name of the protocol by which the file should be accessed, the name of the server that the file is stored on and the pathname of the file on the server, e.g. http://www.healthcentral.co.uk/index.htm (a URL for an HTML file index, accessed by using the Web protocol HTTP).
Virus	Computer terminology – a software program designed to destroy computer data.

	The program enters the computer via a floppy disk or via a network or Internet connection.
Wide area network (WAN)	A computer network extending beyond a hospital or general practice.
Website	One or more linked Web pages accessed through the homepage; the URL of the homepage is made available to users on the Web.
World Wide Web (WWW)	The software, which provides a simple and standard way to find and view documents on the Internet. Developed by CERN, it provides: (a) a standard for the creation of multimedia hypertext documents (HTML); (b) a standard way of giving each document an address on the Internet (URL); and (c) a standard way of transferring documents between computers (HTTP). The Web specification allows formatted text and graphics to be viewed directly by a Web browser and allows other kinds of files to be opened separately by helper applications specified in the Web browser's set-up.
X.400	This is the official international messaging/e-mail standard specified by ITU-TS (International Telecommunications Union). It is less common than the de facto standard SMTP, which looks fit to supplant X.400 in the NHS.

Index